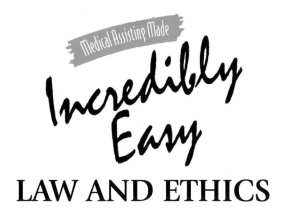

LAW AND ETHICS

D1369537

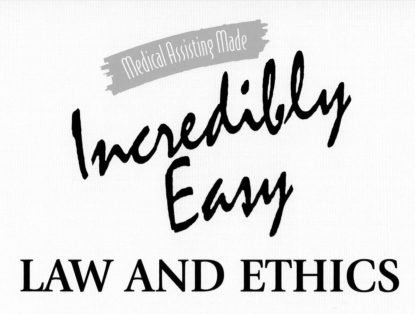

Medical Assisting Made

Incredibly Easy

LAW AND ETHICS

Robyn Gohsman, AAS, RMA, CMAS

Medical Assisting Program
Medical Careers Institute
Newport News, Virginia

Wolters Kluwer | Lippincott Williams & Wilkins
Health
Philadelphia • Baltimore • New York • London
Buenos Aires • Hong Kong • Sydney • Tokyo

Executive Editor: John Goucher
Senior Managing Editor: Rebecca Kerins
Marketing Manager: Nancy Bradshaw
Production Editor: Eve Malakoff-Klein
Illustrator: Bot Roda
Designer: Joan Wendt
Compositor: Circle Graphics, Inc.
Printer: C&C Offset Printing

351 West Camden Street   530 Walnut Street
Baltimore, MD 21201   Philadelphia, PA 19106

Printed in China

9 8 7 6 5 4 3 2 1

Library of Congress Cataloging-in-Publication Data

Gohsman, Robyn.
  Law and ethics / Robyn Gohsman.
    p. ; cm.—(Medical assisting made incredibly easy)
  Includes index.
  ISBN 978-0-7817-7169-6
  1. Medical assistants. 2. Medical ethics. 3. Medical laws and legislation. I. Title. II. Series.
  [DNLM: 1. Ethics, Medical. 2. Legislation, Medical. 3. Allied Health Personnel. 4. Interprofessional Relations. 5. Professional Practice. 6. Professional-Patient Relations. W 33.1 G614L 2009]
  R728.8.G67 2009
  174.2—dc22
                        2007042527

DISCLAIMER

Care has been taken to confirm the accuracy of the information present and to describe generally accepted practices. However, the authors, editors, and publisher are not responsible for errors or omissions or for any consequences from application of the information in this book and make no warranty, expressed or implied, with respect to the currency, completeness, or accuracy of the contents of the publication. Application of this information in a particular situation remains the professional responsibility of the practitioner; the clinical treatments described and recommended may not be considered absolute and universal recommendations.

The authors, editors, and publisher have exerted every effort to ensure that drug selection and dosage set forth in this text are in accordance with the current recommendations and practice at the time of publication. However, in view of ongoing research, changes in government regulations, and the constant flow of information relating to drug therapy and drug reactions, the reader is urged to check the package insert for each drug for any change in indications and dosage and for added warnings and precautions. This is particularly important when the recommended agent is a new or infrequently employed drug.

Some drugs and medical devices presented in this publication have Food and Drug Administration (FDA) clearance for limited use in restricted research settings. It is the responsibility of the health care provider to ascertain the FDA status of each drug or device planned for use in their clinical practice.

To purchase additional copies of this book, call our customer service department at **(800) 638-3030** or fax orders to **(301) 223-2320**. International customers should call **(301) 223-2300**.

Visit Lippincott Williams & Wilkins on the Internet: http://www.lww.com. Lippincott Williams & Wilkins customer service representatives are available from 8:30 am to 6:00 pm, EST.

PREFACE

Medical Assisting Made Incredibly Easy is an exciting new series designed to make learning enjoyable for medical assisting students. Each book in the series uses a light-hearted, humorous approach to presenting information. Maria, a Certified Medical Assistant, guides students through the books, offering helpful tips and insight along the way.

Medical Assisting Made Incredibly Easy takes a practical approach, providing students with the critical information that they need to know, including complete coverage of the core skills they must master in their studies. The series covers all competencies based on the standards and guidelines established for medical assisting by the Commission on Accreditation of Allied Health Educational Programs (CAAHEP) and the Accrediting Bureau of Health Education Schools (ABHES).

About This Book

Medical Assisting Made Incredibly Easy: Law and Ethics provides students with a solid foundation in medical law and ethics, covering essential topics such as the American legal system, risk management and lawsuits, the patient-physician relationship, medical law and statutes, workplace law, medical records and confidentiality, and bioethics. The text covers the Legal Concepts set forth in both CAAHEP's general competencies and in ABHES's competencies. These are among the skills that students must master to pass the test required to become either a Certified Medical Assistant or a Registered Medical Assistant.

Special Features

Medical Assisting Made Incredibly Easy: Law and Ethics is designed to be enjoyable to read, as well as highly informative. Each chapter in this book includes special features designed to guide students in their study. These elements will help students identify the most important information in the chapter and to understand all of it.

- *Chapter Checklist* includes a list of skills and other important information that students will gain after reading the material.

- *Chapter Competencies* highlights the ABHES and CAAHEP competencies covered in each chapter.

- *Legal Brief* summarizes important legal information.

- *By the Book* highlights the medical assistant's impact on ensuring that office operations are carried out according to legal and ethical dictates.

- *Ethics in Action* offers tips about ethics as it pertains to medical assistants.

- *Exhibits* present illustrated examples of concepts presented in the text.

- *What's the Verdict?* presents case studies covering real-life scenarios that medical assistants would need to know how to handle.

- *Letter of the Law* provides a bulleted review of laws that medical assistants need to know.

- *Closing Statements* summarizes a chapter's key content.

- *Before the Bench* tests students on what they have learned via an end-of-chapter quiz.

In addition to the above features, this book also includes bolded key terms throughout each chapter and a Glossary in the back of the book, as well as many other boxed features and tables.

Additional Resources

In addition to the text, the following resources are available for students and instructors:

- An **Online Course** provides interactive exercises and review opportunities that support the text and classroom experience.
- An **Instructor's Resource CD-ROM** with test generator, PowerPoint slides, answers to end-of-chapter quizzes, and customizable competency evaluation forms helps instructors optimize their teaching.
- A complete set of **Lesson Plans** is also available to instructors.

Medical Assisting Made Incredibly Easy: Law and Ethics is designed to make the study of law and ethics fun and effective for medical assisting students. The purpose of this book, and the entire *Medical Assisting Made Incredibly Easy* series, is student success!

USER'S GUIDE

Hello, my name is Maria. I'm a Certified Medical Assistant and educator, as well as your guide through this textbook. There are a number of features in this **Medical Assisting Made Incredibly Easy** text to help you learn everything you need to become a successful medical assistant. Read through this User's Guide to orient yourself to everything the text has to offer. Good luck in your medical assisting studies!

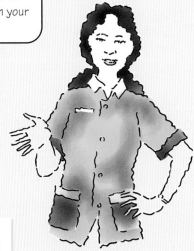

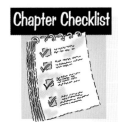

Chapter Checklist

- Explain why a knowledge of law and ethics is important in working in a medical office
- Describe the difference between law, ethics, etiquette, morals, and values
- Distinguish how law and ethics are related
- Compare the consequences of unlawful and unethical behavior
- Recognize the importance of providing good customer service and helping prevent lawsuits

Chapter Checklist orients you to the material that's covered in the current chapter.

Chapter Competencies

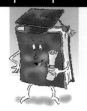

- Perform within legal and ethical boundaries (CAAHEP 3.c.2.b.)
- Demonstrate knowledge of federal and state health care legislation and regulations (CAAHEP 3.c.2.e.)
- Follow established policy in initiating or terminating medical treatment (ABHES 5.d.)

Chapter Competencies tell you which skills are covered in each chapter, as outlined by CAAHEP and ABHES.

Legal Brief DUTY OF CARE AND *RESPONDEAT SUPERIOR*

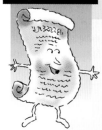

Legal Brief boxes summarize important legal information.

As you learned in Chapter 2, *respondeat superior* is the legal principle that your employer is responsible for your actions if you're acting within your scope of practice. However, *respondeat superior* may not apply if by following the physician's orders you harm a patient, and then you don't let the physician know. Case law has established that failing to tell the physician breaches your duty of care to the patient. If you do not tell the physician, the physician can't correct the situation. For example, a medical assistant instructed to administer an intramuscular injection accidentally hits the sciatic nerve while administering the shot. If the medical assistant lets the patient leave and does not tell the physician, the patient may return to the office due to pain from the shot. In almost every case of this type, the courts have ruled that *both* the employer and the employee must pay damages to the patient.

By the Book STATUTES FOR MEDICAL ASSISTANTS

Two good examples of statutes that will affect your job as a medical assistant are the Controlled Substances Act and the Health Insurance Portability and Accountability Act (HIPAA). Both are federal laws that Congress passed. The Controlled Substances Act regulates how your office handles and prescribes certain drugs. HIPAA sets standards for the privacy of patients' medical records and for the filing of claims to patients' health insurance providers. You'll read much more about these two important laws in later chapters.

By the Book boxes highlight your impact as a medical assistant on ensuring that office operations are carried out according to legal and ethical dictates.

Ethics in Action   A LOOK AT EUTHANASIA

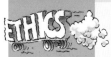

Ethics in Action boxes offer you tips about important ethical issues.

Some patients with terminal illnesses are in great pain. Your compassion can lead you to want to ease their suffering. Some health care workers have helped such patients end their lives by means such as giving enough pain medication to cause death. This is known as **euthanasia.** It makes no difference if the patient consents to "mercy killing" or even begs the health care worker to help him die. In nearly every state, the law views such actions as murder. It's important to behave ethically. But it's also important to obey the law. If your personal values conflict with the law, you must still follow the law every time! If you must, remove yourself from the situation so you do not risk breaking the law.

Exhibits   PATIENT LAWSUITS: WHAT TO EXPECT

Exhibits boxes provide illustrated examples of concepts presented in the text.

The first action in a patient lawsuit starts when the patient files a complaint. The following steps describe what you can expect:

1. If the patient feels that there was a problem with his treatment, the first thing he will do is discuss his concerns with the medical office staff. If he finds the answers acceptable and fair, he might not take legal action. If he still feels there was wrongdoing, he will be on his way to a lawsuit.

What's the Verdict?   AM I GOING TO DIE?

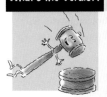

What's the Verdict? boxes present case studies covering real-life scenarios that you'll need to know how to handle.

Charles is a medical assistant in an oncologist's office. (An **oncologist** *is a physician who specializes in treating cancer.) A patient was visibly upset after her treatment as she and Charles arranged an appointment for her next visit. "I'm going to die, aren't I?" she blurted out, as tears welled up in her eyes. Charles knew that patients with her type of cancer have a high cure rate. "Don't worry," he told her. "You're going to be just fine." The comforted patient thanked him and left the office greatly relieved. Did Charles provide an acceptable standard of care in this situation?*

The Verdict: No. Charles acted honestly and openly, but he exceeded his scope of practice by advising the patient about her condition. As a medical assistant, he does not have the education to make such a judgment.

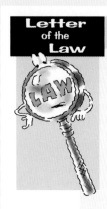

THE CONSUMER PROTECTION ACT

The Consumer Protection Act of 1968 governs payment arrangements that health care providers may make with patients to pay their bills. It requires that the contracts signed by patients must contain the following information:

- total amount for which the patient is responsible
- amount of any down payment the patient has made
- amount of each installment and when it is due
- date of the final payment
- amount of interest, if any, the office is charging the patient

Letter of the Law boxes provide a bulleted review of laws with which medical assistants should be familiar.

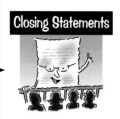

- Medical office employees need to have a good understanding of law and ethics in order to act appropriately, to make decisions in difficult situations, and to provide a high standard of customer service and medical care. Failure to act legally and ethically at all times can lead to lawsuits and loss of income for the office. It can also put you in conflict with the law.

- Laws are rules of conduct that government creates and requires people to obey. Ethics are guidelines for proper behavior that come from other sources than government. The main sources of ethics are personal morals, values, codes of conduct established by professional organizations, and standards that are generally expected by professionals who work in that field.

Closing Statements summarize a chapter's key content.

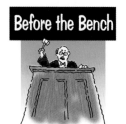

Answer the following multiple-choice questions.

1. The range of activities a medical professional is qualified to perform is called:
   a. scope of practice.
   b. standard of care.
   c. duty of care.
   d. reasonable person standard.

2. According to the AAMA, which of the following is not a common clinical task a medical assistant may be asked to perform?
   a. taking medical histories
   b. removing sutures and changing dressings
   c. performing venipuncture
   d. interpreting test results

Before the Bench provides you with a short quiz so you can test your knowledge.

REVIEWERS

Julie Akason
Argosy University
Eagan, Minnesota

Nina Beaman
Bryant and Stratton College
Richmond, Virginia

Tracie Fuqua
Wallace State Community College
Hanceville, Alabama

Christine Golden
Waukesha County Technical College
Pewaukee, Wisconsin

Kimberly Harrell
Branford Hall Career Institute
Southington, Connecticut

Carolyn Helms
Atlanta Technical College
Atlanta, Georgia

Rebecca Hickey
Butler Technology and Career Development Schools
Fairfield Township, Ohio

Elizabeth Hoffman
Baker College
Clinton Township, Michigan

Joanna Holly
Midstate College
Peoria, Illinois

Helen Houser
Phoenix College
Phoenix, Arizona

Dorothy Kiel
Rhodes State College
Lima, Ohio

Sandra Lehrke
Anoka Technical College
Anoka, Minnesota

Christine Malone
Everett Community College
Everett, Washington

Maureen Messier
Bradford Hall Career Institute
Southington, Connecticut

Lisa Nagle
Augusta Technical College
Augusta, Georgia

Amy Semenchuk
Rockford Business College
Rockford, Illinois

Cheryl Startzell
San Antonio College
San Antonio, Texas

Nina Thierer
Ivy Tech Community College
Fort Wayne, Indiana

Stacey Wilson
Cabarrus College of Health Sciences
Concord, North Carolina

CONTENTS

Chapter 1

INTRODUCING LAW AND ETHICS

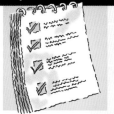

Chapter Checklist

- Explain why a knowledge of law and ethics is important in working in a medical office
- Describe the difference between law, ethics, etiquette, morals, and values
- Distinguish how law and ethics are related
- Compare the consequences of unlawful and unethical behavior
- Recognize the importance of providing good customer service and helping prevent lawsuits

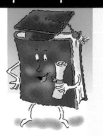

Chapter Competencies

- Identify and respond to issues of confidentiality (CAAHEP 3.c.2.a.)
- Perform within legal and ethical boundaries (CAAHEP 3.c.2.b.)
- Maintain confidentiality at all times (ABHES 1.b.)
- Project a positive attitude (ABHES 1.a.)
- Be cognizant of ethical boundaries (ABHES 1.d.)

Everyone knows that it's important to obey the law. That's fairly easy to understand. But other forces affect our actions, too, and some of them have little to do with the law. Morals, values, ethics, and etiquette also shape our behavior. Also, there are consequences if our behavior falls short in these areas.

The law is usually straightforward. However, sometimes, it can be harder to define what's "right" when it comes to ethics and morals. In this chapter you'll read about the connections and differences between law, ethics, and other forces that determine how we should behave.

What does any of this have to do with work in a medical office? Well, for one thing, you'll be expected to show "proper" behavior on the job. For another, a medical practice's success is closely linked to the actions of its employees. But, most importantly, a good understanding of law and ethics can help make your career as a medical assistant a pleasant and satisfying one.

The Lowdown on Law

Laws are rules of conduct that the government creates and requires us to obey. They ensure that we receive the rights we enjoy as Americans. They also help protect us from being harmed by others. Laws protect us in two ways:

- by prohibiting possibly harmful behaviors or acts
- by discouraging people from committing these acts for fear of punishment

You'll read more about the law and legal system in Chapter 2. But to help you understand why we have laws, think about what life would be like without traffic laws. Suppose there were no speed limits or traffic signals requiring drivers to stop at intersections. How safe would travel be on roads and highways?

Many laws exist to protect the rights and safety of patients. Physicians must abide by certain laws. As a medical assistant, you'll need to have a basic understanding of these laws. It's your responsibility to abide by these laws and to help the physician stay within the boundaries of the law. You may not yet have heard of many of them. But ignorance of the law is no excuse. Just one act of wrongdoing can harm a patient and cause a lawsuit. Knowledge of the laws will help you follow legal guidelines.

Legal Brief PARTNERS IN PROGRESS

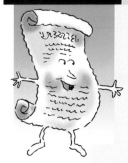

Many patients view themselves as partners with medical professionals in the healing process. This makes them more likely to seek more information about their conditions and to question treatment decisions. Patients expect good outcomes from treatments, especially in light of medical advances and developments. If they are disappointed with the outcome of their treatment, they are much more likely to sue. There are sometimes lawsuits that are initiated not because the physician has done anything wrong, but because patients were dissatisfied with the treatment or support they received from support staff, including medical assistants. This makes your role even more crucial.

As a medical assistant, it's critical that you understand the legal aspects of your relationships with patients. You must be clear about your legal duties and responsibilities regarding patients and their rights. You must also know your role and responsibilities in acting on behalf of the physician. You'll learn about important laws that will affect your work as a medical assistant throughout this book.

All About Ethics

Ethics are guidelines for determining proper behavior. Laws do this, too, but they come from government. Ethics come from two sources.

- **Personal ethics** are guidelines to behavior that result from a person's morals and values.
- **Professional ethics** are standards of conduct that are set by professional organizations or that are generally accepted or expected by the people who work in a field.

MORALS AND VALUES

Morals are a person's ideas about right and wrong. **Values** are principles of worth and importance. Morals and values are closely related. Family and culture influences people's morals and values. **Culture** is a general set of beliefs and behaviors that the people in a society follow. Religion is an important part of culture; it also can be one of the major influences on a person's morals.

- Morals and values are equally important in setting someone's personal ethical standards of conduct.
- In professional ethics, behavior is guided more by values that are generally accepted in the profession.

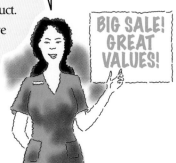

Strong morals and good values are the keys to ethical behavior.

BIG SALE! GREAT VALUES!

MEDICAL ETHICS

Medical ethics are principles of conduct that govern the behavior of health care professionals. They focus on the rights, welfare, and concerns of patients. Medical ethics will affect your professional ethics as a medical assistant.

As there are more advances in the medical field, there are more ethical boundaries that must be explored. **Bioethics** deals with moral issues and questions that arise from advances in medicine and in the biological and health sciences. Some current bioethics issues involve:

- questions of when life begins
- the morality of genetic engineering
- the ethics of stem cell research

When it comes to bioethical issues, religion and culture often play a significant role in what individuals believe to be right or wrong. This is especially the case with topics including stem cell research and abortion. As a medical assistant, it's important that you're aware and sensitive when dealing with such issues. You'll read more about bioethics in Chapter 10.

No medical professional can be successful for long if his conduct toward patients, physicians, or coworkers is unethical. Medical ethics determines medical customs, proper behavior in medical settings and situations, and professional courtesy. For example, stealing medications or prescription pads from the physician is not only illegal but unethical as well.

VALUES AND ETHICS

A person's values play an important role in how he or she acts. You may call on your own values when determining proper behavior in a professional setting. You'll read more later about

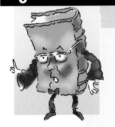

By the Book   ETHICAL BEHAVIOR IN THE MEDICAL OFFICE

Work in a medical office can sometimes require behavior that may be contrary to your personal ethics. For example, suppose a patient doesn't want her family to know about her health problem. Personally, you feel strongly that her loved ones deserve to know. However, you must not violate her legal right to privacy. This is just one example that shows why professional ethics are usually a better guide for office behavior than your personal views of right and wrong.

how values shape professional ethics in medical assistants. But there are also values that are important to people who show high standards in their personal behavior.

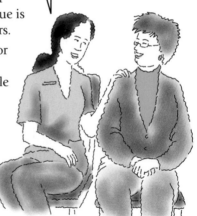

Wanting to help others is a personal value of mine. It makes me a better health care professional!

- **Beneficence** means doing good, especially doing things that will benefit other people. Someone who possesses this value is caring and concerned with helping others.
- Another value that affects personal behavior is **humility,** or showing modesty in your opinion of your own importance. A humble person doesn't think of himself as more important than someone else.

By having strong personal values, you'll find that it will be easier to behave correctly in a professional setting. And these personal values will not go unnoticed by your supervisors and staff. The physician will appreciate your contributions toward the success of her practice, and you'll benefit from great opportunities on the job.

UP WITH PEOPLE

One sure sign of ethical behavior is that it shows respect and concern for others. The values discussed above focus more on other people than they do on the person who holds them.

But even values that don't appear to focus primarily on other people actually do. For example, look at the value of **responsibility.**

Ethics in Action   CONSIDERING ETIQUETTE

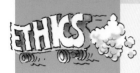

Etiquette is rules of polite behavior. You can think of etiquette as courtesy or good manners. The rules of etiquette can vary. Some behaviors that are appropriate in one culture may be bad manners in another. For instance, in some Asian cultures, waving hello is impolite. In Western cultures, it's a sign of friendship.

In nearly every profession, there are standards of etiquette for how members treat one another and expect to be treated themselves. For example, in the medical profession, it's common courtesy to address physicians with the title "doctor" before their last name. It's also important to address your patients appropriately. This may mean referring to the patient as "Mrs. Smith" in some areas or "Sue Smith" in other cases. Check with your supervisor on how you should address patients.

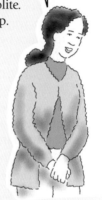
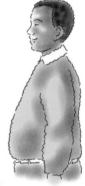

Proper etiquette, including saying please and thank you, can go a long way in developing good patient relationships.

Showing responsibility means being dependable and willing to accept the consequences of your actions. Acting responsibly means that you don't blame other people if something goes wrong. We all make mistakes, but it shows responsibility to admit when you've made a mistake and to take corrective action. Like beneficence and humility, responsibility shows that you consider other people's situations and feelings as important as your own.

Never forget that professional ethics require you to put other people's interests ahead of your own. In most professions, that means putting customers first. In health care, patients are the customers. Medical ethics require that medical professionals *always* put what's best for the patient ahead of all other concerns. If you don't, you could be fired or sued.

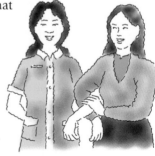

Don't lose sight of the fact you're there because the patient is there. No patients = no job!

Brothers But Not Twins

Learning and applying the principles of law and ethics can be complicated. The two subjects are closely related. At the same time, they are different in many ways.

For example, ethics often shapes behavior before laws do. Discrimination is a good example. Racial and gender discrimination were moral issues for some people long before laws made them illegal.

> One difference between law and ethics is that unethical behavior can get you fired and unlawful behavior can get you arrested!

LEGAL AND ETHICAL LIMITS

Another difference is that laws are more limited than ethics. That's because most legal standards are negative. Behaving lawfully often involves *not* doing something.

Laws forbid us to harm people, but they usually don't require us to help them. It's illegal to rob someone, but no law requires you to call the police if you see someone being robbed. Ethical standards are more positive. Many people's ethics would cause them to call the police. Their morals would tell them it's the right thing to do.

Other people believe that they have no responsibility beyond obeying the law. They believe that a behavior is "wrong" only if the law forbids it. But there are times when behaving lawfully is not necessarily acting ethically. Lying is one example. There's no law against lying, but most people would consider it unethical. As a medical assistant, you'll encounter similar situations. That's just one more reason why understanding ethics is so important.

ETHICAL DILEMMAS

This overlap of law and ethics can be confusing. As you just read, a behavior or action may be unethical, but it still may be legal. In other words, not all unethical acts are illegal. Again, lying is a good example.

On the other hand, most illegal acts are also unethical. Some illegal acts *can* be ethical, however. For example, although it's illegal to break into someone's home, it would be ethical to do so if an injured person inside needed help.

To make things even more complicated, as you've already read, personal ethics and professional ethics can sometimes clash. When ethics and law—or ethical standards—differ, a dilemma can result. A **dilemma** is a problem caused by a conflict between choices. In an ethical dilemma, the conflict is between rights, responsibilities, and values. See the "Exhibits" feature on page 8 for an example of an ethical dilemma.

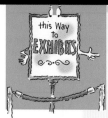

Exhibits

RESOLVING ETHICAL DILEMMAS

Dilemmas require tough choices. Sometimes, you may not know what the ethical action should be. At other times, you may believe that your choice of action is right, but for some reason you may hesitate to act on it.

Consider the following. Suppose you work for a family physician in a small town. He has been serving the community for over 40 years. He is now 70 years old and beginning to show signs of dementia. He forgets to review patient test results and has also seemed disoriented and confused on several occasions. You respect the physician and are hesitant to question his abilities. But, at the same time, you also know that patients deserve high-quality care. You're concerned that the physician's behavior may be affecting patient safety. Do you protect the physician's license by keeping your thoughts to yourself? Or do you ensure patient safety by reporting your concerns to your supervisor, the physician himself, or even the state board of medicine? That's an ethical dilemma!

Here's a process that will help you decide what to do in an ethical dilemma.

1. Make sure that you fully understand the situation that's causing the dilemma.

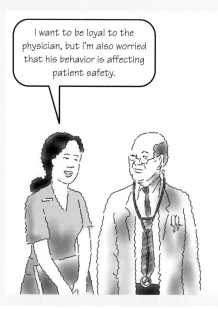

2. List your range of choices for action and examine each one. For each choice, first determine if it's legal. If it's not, eliminate it as a choice.

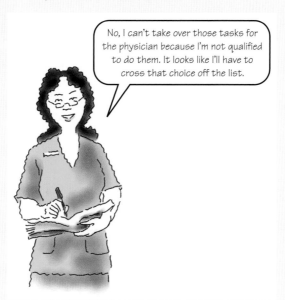

No, I can't take over those tasks for the physician because I'm not qualified to do them. It looks like I'll have to cross that choice off the list.

3. Determine the likely result of each action on each of the parties affected by the situation. For example, you might decide to speak to the office manager or the physician directly before contacting the state board.

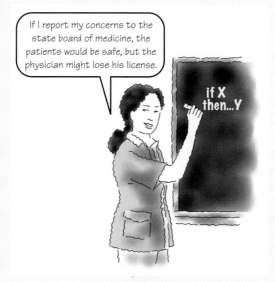

If I report my concerns to the state board of medicine, the patients would be safe, but the physician might lose his license.

if X then...Y

4. For each choice, ask yourself if the harm done to some of the parties will be greater than the good done for others.

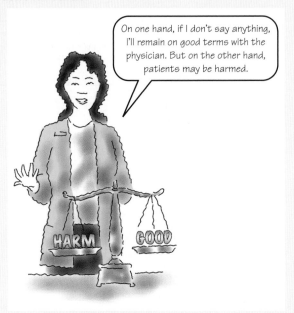

Following these steps will make the ethics of each choice clearer and the right decision much easier to understand.

Ethics for Medical Assistants

Imagine that you're having dinner in a restaurant. The waitstaff ignore you and appear unconcerned that you might be hungry. They respond rudely when you ask questions about the menu. When they bring your food, it's not what you ordered. During the meal, you have to ask to get your water glass refilled, and you have a hard time getting anyone's attention.

The food was excellent, but how likely are you to go back to that restaurant when the service was so inattentive and unprofessional? How likely would you be to recommend that restaurant to other people?

Now imagine that the restaurant was actually a medical office, and that the waitstaff were medical assistants. Imagine that the restaurants' customers, like you, were patients. Ask yourself the same questions: Would you go back to that medical office? Would you recommend it to others?

If the staff of a medical office acts unprofessionally, some customers (patients) aren't likely to return, no matter how good the physician is. When enough patients are unhappy about their experience or have heard about another patient's bad experience, you won't have many more "customers" walking through the door.

No patients, no paycheck!

PROFESSIONAL ETHICS

As a medical assistant, your behavior must meet certain standards. This is important if you and your office are going to provide good customer service. But it's even more important to comply with the medical profession's ethical standards.

At the very minimum, medical ethics require that you:

- protect the privacy of patient information
- follow all state and federal laws
- be honest in all your actions

You must always follow ethical standards as you perform your duties. As you've already read, medical ethics require that your concern and focus always be on the rights, welfare, and concerns of patients. This means that you should show all patients the same kindness and respect.

At the same time, you must never share your personal opinions about medical issues with them. You also must ignore your personal feelings of right and wrong in dealing with patients. For example, if you believe that sexual relations between unmarried persons is immoral, you must not let your feelings affect how you treat single women seeking information about birth control.

Codes of Ethics

Many professional groups write codes of ethics to help their members behave ethically. The American Association of Medical Assistants (AAMA) is one of the two national professional organizations for medical assistants. It has created five guidelines for medical assistants to follow.

1. Provide services with respect for human dignity.
2. Respect patient confidentiality, except when information is required by law.

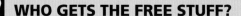

What's the Verdict? WHO GETS THE FREE STUFF?

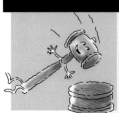

A salesman for a drug company leaves a large supply of prescription allergy medicine sample packets with an office's medical assistant. The date by which the packets should be used is about to expire. Members of the office staff ask the medical assistant to give them some of the packets for their own use. Should the medical assistant grant their request?

The Verdict: Good question! This is actually a double-whammy when it comes to law and ethics. It would be both unethical and illegal for the medical assistant to give these free samples to co-workers unless told to do so by the physician. Drug company representatives leave free samples for the physician to give to patients. Even if all the packets may not be given away before they expire, professional ethics require that the medical assistant put the welfare of the office's patients ahead of coworkers' desire for free medication. And because it's a prescription medication, it can't be dispensed without the physician's orders. It would be illegal for a medical assistant to distribute prescription medicine without a license.

3. Uphold the honor and high principles set forth by the AAMA.
4. Continually improve knowledge and skills for the benefit of patients and the health care team.
5. Take part in community services and activities that promote good health and welfare to the general public.

Confidentiality

Patient confidentiality is one of the most important ethical principles a medical assistant must observe. In Chapter 7, you'll learn about the laws that dictate when a patient's medical information can and can't be released.

Say "No" to Secrets

Any interactions with a patient are confidential, including your conversations and treatment. Patients will often reveal some of their innermost feelings, thoughts, and fears to their medical caregivers. Remember that this information is not for public knowledge.

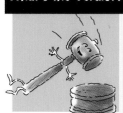

What's the Verdict? KEEPING A SECRET

A patient tells me that she has been feeling really down lately and finds herself crying frequently. She has started taking some of her husband's antidepressants to make herself feel better. She asks me not to tell the doctor because she knows he will tell her that she should get some help and go for some counseling. She doesn't think that's necessary. What should I do?

The Verdict: Occasionally, patients will reveal their innermost feelings, thoughts, and fears to their medical assistant. And sometimes they may ask that you *not* share this information with the physician. However, you are legally and ethically obligated to share all patient information with the physician—it's your job. So, in this case, you can't keep the patient's secret. You should tell the patient that you have to tell the physician any information that she shares with you in the medical office. You should also remind her that it's in her best interest for you to share this information with the physician. The physician is in the best position to provide necessary care and will know how to proceed.

All in the Family

Family members, clergy, and friends may want to know how a patient is doing. These questions are almost always asked with good intentions. However, it's both illegal and unethical to answer them without the patient's consent.

THE "VALUED" MEDICAL ASSISTANT

As you've learned, the most important value in any medical office is a commitment to putting patients first. This behavior is equally true for medical assistants. Your most important responsibility will be to place the patient's best interests first at all times. To do otherwise is highly unethical.

You've already read about some of the other values that shape ethical behavior. These are all important to ethical behavior in a medical office too. For example, are you familiar with the oath physicians take that

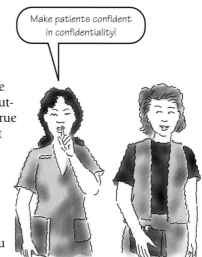

Make patients confident in confidentiality!

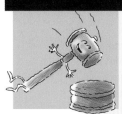

What's the Verdict?

TO TELL OR NOT TO TELL?

A patient's lab tests show that he has a sexually transmitted disease. He begs the medical assistant to say nothing to his wife about his test result. He says, "My marriage will be ruined if she finds out I've been unfaithful!" The medical assistant knows the wife needs to be tested—and treated if she's contracted the disease. Should the medical assistant say something to the wife?

The Verdict: Whether the patient asks that his secret be kept or not, the medical assistant must not say anything to the wife. The law may require that the positive test result be reported to the health department. But it's up to the health department to contact the patient's sexual partners. Professional ethics requires the medical assistant to respect patient confidentiality.

states, "First do no harm"? Beneficence is the value expressed in this oath. As a medical assistant, you'll be representing the physician in many situations. Therefore, this standard of ethical behavior applies to you, too.

Empathize, Don't Sympathize

It's important to have empathy for patients. **Empathy** is imagining, understanding, and being sensitive to another person's experiences, thoughts, and feelings. Think of having empathy for others as putting yourself "in their shoes." However, empathy should not be confused with **sympathy,** which is feeling pity for someone. It's easy to feel sorry for patients sometimes, especially if they're suffering. But most patients will react better to someone who has empathy for them instead. It's important to show understanding for their situation, feelings, and views without feeling sorry for them. You should never say to a patient, "I know what you're going through!"

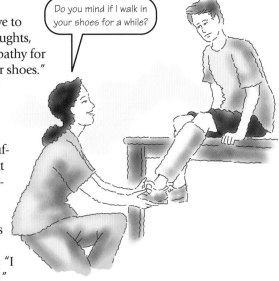

Do you mind if I walk in your shoes for a while?

Professionalism and Personality

A medical assistant needs to exhibit personality as well as professionalism in the medical office. Acting professionally keeps you focused on ethical and legal standards of care. Being friendly makes your dealings with patients easier. It also makes patients feel like you know them, respect them, and care about them.

It's helpful to review the patient's chart prior to his visit. This will help remind you about each particular patient and the information in the chart. For example, if there's a note in the patient's chart from the last visit that said he was preparing to go on a cruise, ask how the trip was. Patients are very impressed when you show this kind of interest in them.

If you don't have specific questions, simply ask patients how they're feeling or if you can do anything else for them. They will remember that you went out of your way to help them, whether it was listening to their concerns or speaking in a kind manner. A cheerful, warm, and professional attitude will be a big help in doing your job.

Show Your Fidelity

Fidelity is faithfulness and loyalty to others. Professional ethics require you to perform your duties in a way that shows loyalty to your employer. But you have to be careful here. If your employer wants you do to something that is harmful to patients or is illegal or unethical in some other way, fidelity does *not* require you to do as the physician asked.

Oops, I Made a Mistake

Showing **honesty** means that you're truthful in every situation. Honesty is an especially important value in professional ethics in the medical field. You must have the personal strength of character to admit you made an error. For example, if you give the wrong medication to a patient, you must notify your supervisor or the physician immediately.

In the medical profession, failing to admit mistakes can have very serious results, including great harm to patients and possible lawsuits. If you're not able to admit your mistakes, you should think about working in another field besides medicine.

How High Are Your Standards?

People with integrity are dedicated to maintaining high standards. **Integrity** is the quality of strongly sticking to your principles. For example, having integrity means that you wash your hands after all contact with every patient, even if no one is looking.

Ethics in Action   THE MEDICAL ASSISTANT'S CREED

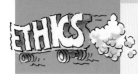

The AAMA Medical Assistant Creed focuses on integrity, fidelity, and other important values of professional ethics. Using the creed as a guide in working with patients and coworkers will help you act in an ethical manner.

- I believe in the principles and purposes of the profession of medical assisting.
- I endeavor to be more effective.
- I aspire to render greater service.
- I protect the confidence entrusted to me.
- I am dedicated to the care and well-being of all people.
- I am loyal to my employer.
- I am true to the ethics of my profession.
- I am strengthened by compassion, courage, and faith.

Dependability and integrity go hand in hand. Another way you can show integrity is by being on time for work each day and not abusing your time at work. Once you arrive at work, you should be working. This means not tending to personal matters during the workday. You should leave personal matters such as phone calls until breaks, lunchtime, or even your day off.

> You may have to make several attempts before you're successful in getting the answers you need. Be persistent.

Justice for All

Justice is fairness in your actions toward all people. You behave justly when you apply the same rules to everyone. Another closely related value is **tolerance,** which means showing respect for people with opinions, beliefs, practices, or backgrounds that are different from your own. It's part of your ethical duty to show all patients the same kindness and respect, regardless of your personal feelings and opinions about them.

I Will Persevere

Health care can be a demanding field to work in. **Perseverance,** or continuing with an action despite obstacles, is a desirable value for a medical assistant. It means that you're likely to get the job done, even when it's difficult.

The Responsible Road

Responsibility is closely related to honesty and integrity. As you read earlier, it means being willing to answer for your actions, whether they were right or wrong. It also means that you can be depended on to do your job and to do it correctly. Responsibility is a sign of maturity in an employee.

STRIVE FOR EXCELLENCE

The duties of your position as a medical assistant will give you a high profile with patients. You'll be an important patient contact and provider of care. Professional ethics exist to guide you as you do this work. Professional ethics keep you focused on proper behavior and on providing outstanding customer service and care.

Behaving ethically shows dedication to your profession. Dedication to the standards of medical ethics will make you a model of excellence for patients, for your coworkers, and within the medical assisting community. Remember that your actions and words all reflect your values, ethics, and dedication to the profession of medical assisting.

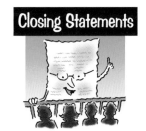

Closing Statements

- Medical office employees need to have a good understanding of law and ethics in order to act appropriately, to make decisions in difficult situations, and to provide a high standard of customer service and medical care. Failure to act legally and ethically at all times can lead to lawsuits and loss of income for the office. It can also put you in conflict with the law.

- Laws are rules of conduct that government creates and requires people to obey. Ethics are guidelines for proper behavior that come from other sources than government. The main sources of ethics are personal morals, values, codes of conduct established by professional organizations, and standards that are generally expected by professionals who work in that field.

- Morals are a person's ideas about right and wrong, while values are generally accepted principles of importance and worth. Both may result from the influences of the person's family and culture. Rules for polite behavior are called etiquette. Like values and morals, etiquette is determined by culture.

- Law and ethics overlap but are not identical. Some behaviors that are legal may be unethical. However, nearly all behaviors that are illegal are unethical, too.

- Unethical behaviors can cause a medical professional to be fired. Illegal behaviors can lead to a medical professional's arrest. Both types of behaviors can result in lawsuits.

- Medical assistants who perform their duties in a legal and ethical manner show high levels of professionalism, provide good customer service, and reduce the possibility that lawsuits will result from their actions.

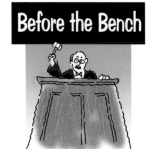

Before the Bench

Answer the following multiple-choice questions.

1. Laws and ethics are alike because they:
   a. are created by government.
   b. guide people's behavior.
   c. are based on morals and values.
   d. determine people's values.

2. Who is the *most* likely to be punished?
   a. someone who breaks a law
   b. someone with low morals
   c. someone who behaves unethically
   d. someone who violates a code of conduct

3. A person's values help determine:
   a. whether the person's actions are illegal.
   b. the person's morals.
   c. how the person behaves.
   d. the person's family and culture.

4. Behaviors that are unethical:
   a. may not be against the law.
   b. are acceptable to most people.
   c. always lead to ethical dilemmas.
   d. can sometimes still be proper.

5. Which of the following is *not* part of medical ethics?
   a. laws that govern the practice of medicine
   b. values that are considered important in health care
   c. proper etiquette in the medical community
   d. personal morals of health care workers

6. Etiquette is *mainly* determined by:
   a. law.
   b. culture.
   c. values.
   d. morals.

7. What is the *most* important requirement of professional ethics for a medical assistant?
   a. Don't do anything you personally believe to be wrong.
   b. Keep current on your skills and knowledge of the law.
   c. Keep the patient's family fully informed and up to date.
   d. Always put the patient's rights and welfare first.

8. Unethical behavior in a medical office is likely to lead to:
   a. poor customer service.
   b. fewer patients for the practice.
   c. lawsuits.
   d. all of the above

9. If a patient asks for a service that you believe is morally wrong, you should:
   a. keep your opinion to yourself.
   b. make sure the physician knows how you feel.
   c. refuse to pass the request on to the physician.
   d. try to talk the patient out of making the request.

10. Which value or behavior is important to helping a medical assistant provide good customer service to patients?
   a. fidelity
   b. empathy
   c. sympathy
   d. all of the above

Chapter 2

LAW IN THE USA

Chapter Checklist

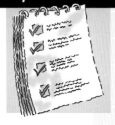

- Define the three main sources of law

- Describe the three different types of law

- Compare and contrast criminal and civil law

- Define *respondeat superior* and explain how it relates in a health care setting

- Identify the three parts of a valid contract

- Differentiate between expressed and implied contracts

- List the steps a physician must follow when terminating a contract

- List the steps of the litigation process, including the roles of the parties or individuals involved

Chapter Competencies

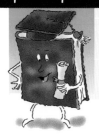

- Perform within legal and ethical boundaries (CAAHEP 3.c.2.b.)

- Demonstrate knowledge of federal and state health care legislation and regulations (CAAHEP 3.c.2.e.)

- Follow established policy in initiating or terminating medical treatment (ABHES 5.d.)

At some point in your career as a medical assistant, your employer may be involved in a lawsuit. You may even be involved yourself—either as a witness or as the result of something you did or failed to do. Or, your employer may ask you to provide records to the court or to attorneys for one side or the other. In any case, a lawsuit can be a frightening thing. The good news is that knowledge of the law can help reduce that fear. This chapter will provide you with a basic knowledge of the law and the legal system, as well as describe what to expect if your office is ever sued.

> Let's see, we've got a legislative branch, an executive branch, and a judicial branch. Just what kind of tree is this?

Where Do Laws Come From?

As you learned in Chapter 1, a good way to understand the law is to think of it as a large set of rules within which we all live. These rules come from three places.

- Legislative bodies enact them.
- Government agencies create them.
- Cases tried in courts of law produce them.

You may have noticed that the three sources of law are the same as the three branches of American government:

- legislative branch
- executive branch
- judicial branch

THE LEGISLATIVE BRANCH

The legislative branch is the arm of government that is mainly responsible for making laws.

- In the federal government, the legislative branch is the U.S. Congress.
- In state government, the state legislature is the legislative branch.
- In cities and towns, the city or town council is the legislative branch of government.

Congress is the most important of the three legislative levels. No law passed by a state legislature can replace or contradict a law passed by Congress. In general, laws passed by a city or town council can't replace or contradict laws passed by that state's legislature. And they can never replace or contradict laws passed by Congress. This makes the laws that Congress passes, which are called **federal laws,** the most powerful laws in the land.

THE EXECUTIVE BRANCH

The executive branch is responsible for enforcing the laws passed by the legislative branch. At each level of government, the executive branch is headed by a chief executive.

- The president of the United States is the chief executive of the federal government.
- The state governor is the chief executive of each state's executive branch.
- The mayor heads the executive branch of city and town governments.

At each level of government, the executive branch consists of agencies or departments that enforce certain laws. One good example is a city's police department, which enforces traffic laws and many other statutes. Another example of an executive agency is a state's medical licensing board. Its job is to enforce the state's medical practice act. Still another example is the U.S. Drug Enforcement Administration (DEA), which helps to enforce the nation's drug laws.

Executive branch agencies often create rules and regulations that help enforce the laws. These rules and regulations also make the laws clearer to those who must abide by them. This helps people avoid breaking the law. You'll read more about rules and regulations later in this chapter.

THE JUDICIAL BRANCH

The courts make up the judicial branch of government. Their job is to interpret and apply the law. In other words, the courts determine what a law means and decide whether someone who has been accused of breaking the law has actually done so.

Each level of government also has a judicial branch. A case may be heard by a local court, a state court, or a federal count, depending on the type of law involved. For example, a local court will hear the case of a person accused of a traffic offense. But if the person is charged with a federal crime, such as Medicare fraud, the case will be tried in federal court.

In addition, courts can actually make laws. You'll see how this happens when you read about the types of law next.

Understanding the Three Sources of Law

Branch of Government	What They Do	Types of Law Produced
Legislative Branch 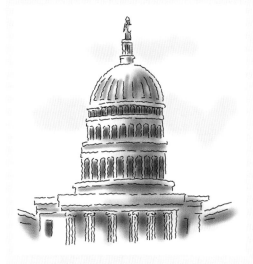	The legislative branches make the laws for the country, state, and cities or towns. Congress is the most important law-making body in the legislative branch. Congress passes federal laws that are the most powerful in the country.	The legislative branch creates statutory law.
Executive Branch 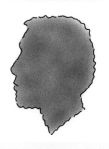	The executive branch enforces the laws passed by the legislative branch. Each level of government has a chief executive who is responsible for seeing that the laws are properly followed. These chief executives include the president of the United States, state governors, and mayors.	Government agencies in the executive branch create administrative law.
Judicial Branch 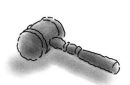	The judicial branch is made up of the courts that interpret and apply the law. There are federal, state, and local courts.	The courts in the judicial branch are responsible for case law.

Three Types of Law

Each branch of government produces a different kind of law.

- Statutory law comes from the legislative branch.
- The executive branch creates administrative law.
- Case law results from the actions of the judicial branch.

> Understanding the basics makes the legal system seem less intimidating and helps protect your patients, your employer, and yourself.

STATUTORY LAW

The laws passed by Congress or by state legislatures are called **statutes.** Laws passed at the local level—for example, by a city council—are called ordinances. Taken together, statutes and ordinances form a body of law known as **statutory law.** Statutes are the main type of statutory law that will affect your work as a medical assistant.

Statutes begin as bills that are introduced into Congress or your state's legislature by one of its members. If the legislature passes the bill, it becomes a law—unless the president or state governor vetoes, or rejects, it. However, if a bill is vetoed, a legislature can sometimes pass the bill again and make it law anyway.

Once it has been passed, a law can be changed or replaced by another law. It can also be repealed, which means it is officially withdrawn as a law. Individuals also may challenge the law in court as being a violation of the state or U.S. Constitution.

By the Book — STATUTES FOR MEDICAL ASSISTANTS

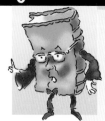

Two good examples of statutes that will affect your job as a medical assistant are the Controlled Substances Act and the Health Insurance Portability and Accountability Act (HIPAA). Both are federal laws that Congress passed. The Controlled Substances Act regulates how your office handles and prescribes certain drugs. HIPAA sets standards for the privacy of patients' medical records and for the filing of claims to patients' health insurance providers. You'll read much more about these two important laws in later chapters.

ADMINISTRATIVE LAW

A government agency creates **administrative law.** Because administrative laws are not passed by legislatures, they are not statutes. Instead, they are called **administrative rules** or **regulations.** Violation of these laws can be considered as serious an offense as breaking a statutory law.

The main purpose of administrative law is to provide details that make statutes more clear. For example, a state's medical practices statute may require a physician to be a graduate of an accredited medical school. What exactly does that mean? Accredited by whom? Many groups rate and approve medical schools. In this case, the state medical board would create an administrative rule, or regulation, specifying the accreditation needed for a medical school's graduates to be licensed in that state.

Another good example is HIPAA. The statute requires that a patient's privacy be protected, but Congress authorized a U.S. government agency, the U.S. Department of Health and Human Services (HHS), to create regulations about how that can be done. The procedures you follow when you handle patients' records in the office are probably based on HHS regulations, which are part of administrative law. Breaking one of these regulations is also a violation of HIPAA, the statutory authority behind the regulations.

REVERE THE CONSTITUTION

The U.S. Constitution is the highest law of the land. No statute or other law may limit or deny a right, freedom, or power that is granted in the Constitution. Determining if a law does this is a job of the courts. However, courts do not automatically review laws to see if they violate the Constitution. Someone affected by a law first must bring a case, charging that the law is unconstitutional. Whatever decision the court reaches, the law's supporters may appeal the decision to a higher court for review.

The U.S. Supreme Court has the final word on whether a state or federal law violates the U.S. Constitution. A state's supreme court has the final word on whether a state law violates that state's constitution.

CASE LAW

The courts of the judicial branch are the third source of law. When judges decide cases, they first look at previous cases tried under the same law to determine how the law was applied.

Those earlier decisions become **precedents,** or guides, that the judge applies in deciding the current case.

The legal principle is called *stare decisis,* which is Latin for "let the decision stand." It means that decisions in current court cases are based on decisions in similar past cases. Because this type of law comes from past court cases rather than from legislatures or government agencies, it's known as **case law.** It's also called **common law,** because it applies in all situations for which the facts are the same.

> It's okay to be unoriginal when you're dealing with legal precedents. That's what *stare decisis* is all about!

ENGLISH COMMON LAW

The first common law came from decisions made by judges in English courts about 800 years ago. The English colonists brought this body of law to America in the 1600s. But life on the American frontier was very different than in England. Some of the old common law precedents didn't fit the conditions in the colonies. So, colonial courts made decisions that set new precedents. This caused the body of common law to grow in America.

Common law continues to grow and change as new conditions require new precedents. Every state except Louisiana follows English common law. In Louisiana, which was first colonized by France, common law is based on early French law.

A good example of common law is a physician's duty to provide good care to a patient. This requirement is hardly ever stated in a statute or in administrative law. But decisions in court cases have established that it's a physician's professional responsibility to provide good care. This makes it a legal requirement for physicians under common law.

Public Law and Private Law

You just read that there are three types of law—statutory law, administrative law, and case law—depending on who makes the law. There is also another way of looking at the law: by whom or what it applies to, rather than its origin. Looking at the law this way identifies two broad divisions of law.

* **Public law** is law that affects everyone. The most common type of public law is **criminal law.** Although crimes are

Legal Brief   BUT IT WAS AN ACCIDENT . . .

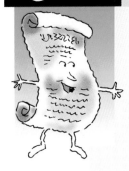

If your actions harm a patient, you're legally responsible—even if you didn't intend to cause harm. This principle of common law was established all the way back in 1616, in the case of *Weaver v. Ward*.

Weaver and Ward were both soldiers. Ward accidentally fired his musket during training. The musket ball hit Weaver, who happened to be standing nearby. Weaver sued Ward. The judge decided the case in Weaver's favor. He said that, because Ward didn't shoot Weaver on purpose, Ward had not committed a crime. However, he ruled that Weaver had a right not to be injured by Ward's action, even if it was an accident. So Weaver had to pay Ward for accidentally harming him.

committed against individuals, criminal law exists to protect all of society.

- **Civil law** involves relationships between individuals, or between a person and the government. For this reason, civil law is also sometimes called **private law.**

At first, these different ways of viewing the law may seem contradictory. But they really are not. That's because some statutory, administrative, and case laws are classified as criminal law, and others are classified as civil law.

Although both types of law are equally important to our legal system, you'll primarily read about civil law in this chapter, because it has a greater effect on your daily work as a medical assistant.

CRIMINAL OR CIVIL LAW?

Violations of criminal law are often violations of civil law, too. For example, murder is a crime. The accused murderer will have a criminal trial, and he probably will go to prison if found guilty. In addition, under civil law, the murder victim's family can sue the accused murderer for wrongful death. He would then also have to pay money to the victim's family if found guilty in a separate civil trial.

CRIMINAL LAW

Crimes are violations of criminal law. These violations can occur in either of two ways:

- when someone takes an action that's been banned, such as driving while drunk
- when someone fails to take an action that's required, such as failing to stop for a red light at an intersection

There are two types of crimes.

- **Felonies** are serious crimes that are punishable by long prison sentences or even by death. Some of the more notorious felonies include murder, rape, kidnapping, robbery, and arson.
- **Misdemeanors** are less serious crimes that are punishable by fines or short jail sentences. Examples include traffic offenses, stealing something worth a small amount of money, and disturbing the peace.

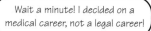

Wait a minute! I decided on a medical career, not a legal career!

Crime in the Medical Office

Although it's unlikely that you'll be involved with any crimes in your work as a medical assistant, they can and do sometimes occur. This section includes examples of crimes that you might encounter in a medical office.

Abuse

Child abuse is a felony and one of the leading causes of death in children under the age of five years. According to federal law, child abuse is any act or failure to act by a parent or caregiver that results in the death or serious emotional or physical harm of a child, including sexual abuse and exploitation. Those actions that put a child at risk of death or harm are also considered abuse. The federal Child Abuse Prevention and Treatment Act mandates that threats to a child's physical and mental welfare be reported. State laws vary regarding the procedure for reporting abuse. However, as a medical assistant, you're professionally and ethically responsible for reporting any suspected abuse to the physician. She will know how to proceed. This applies not only to child abuse, but also to spousal abuse and elder abuse. You'll read more about this subject in Chapter 6.

Embezzlement

Embezzlement is wrongfully taking money or property that you're responsible for and using it for your own personal needs.

An employee who steals money from his employer is committing embezzlement, which is a felony.

Fraud

Fraud is any deceitful act with the intention of concealing the truth. Submitting a claim that you know to be false to a patient's health insurance plan is one example of fraud. Falsifying medical records can also be considered fraud in some cases. Fraud is a felony, too.

Battery

Battery is the actual physical touching of a person without her consent. This can range from acts such as striking an employee or a patient to various kinds of sexual contact. All acts are felonies.

Accessory to Crime

If you're aware of a crime and do nothing about it, your lack of action is also a criminal act. An **accessory** is someone who does not actually commit the crime, but who directly or indirectly contributes to it. Here are some behaviors that could cause someone to be charged as an accessory to a crime:

- encouraging another person to commit a crime
- witnessing a crime and doing nothing
- helping cover up a crime after it has been committed

> Practicing medicine without a license is a felony. That's one reason you should never treat a patient without a physician's order.

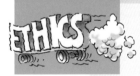

Ethics in Action   A LOOK AT EUTHANASIA

Some patients with terminal illnesses are in great pain. Your compassion can lead you to want to ease their suffering. Some health care workers have helped such patients end their lives by means such as giving enough pain medication to cause death. This is known as **euthanasia.** It makes no difference if the patient consents to "mercy killing" or even begs the health care worker to help him die. In nearly every state, the law views such actions as murder. It's important to behave ethically. But it's also important to obey the law. If your personal values conflict with the law, you must still follow the law every time! If you must, remove yourself from the situation so you do not risk breaking the law.

What's the Verdict?   AN ACCESSORY TO FRAUD

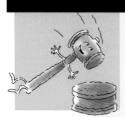

One of your coworkers is billing for services the physician never provided to bring more money into the practice. You learn about this accidentally while reviewing bills. You know it's a clear case of fraud, but how do you handle the situation? You get along with this coworker and don't want to cause problems in the office.

The Verdict: According to the law, you must report it immediately. If you don't, you would be helping your coworker cover up fraud. You could be criminally charged as an accessory to the crime. Even if you're friendly with this coworker, you must prioritize your ethics and professionalism to protect your office and yourself from further legal problems.

> Accessories can make a great wardrobe, but you want to avoid being an accessory in the medical office!

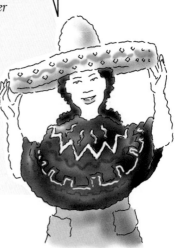

Criminal Court Cases

A person is accused of a crime when charges are brought by the local, state, or federal government. The level of government bringing the charges depends on whether the person is accused of breaking a local, state, or federal law.

Defendants and Plaintiffs

The person accused of breaking the law is called the **defendant.** The party that charges the wrongdoing is called the **plaintiff.**

Legal Brief   NAME THAT COURT CASE!

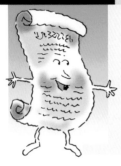

All original court cases are titled by listing the name of the plaintiff first and then the name of the defendant. For example, a criminal case might be called *United States v. John Doe* if the plaintiff is the federal government. (The abbreviation "v." stands for "versus.") In a state or local criminal case, the plaintiff might be listed as the state or as simply "The People"—for example, *The People v. John Doe,* or *Ohio v. John Doe.*

Because in criminal cases the government is the plaintiff, the plaintiff is also called the **prosecution.**

The Attorneys

An attorney usually represents each side in a court case. In a criminal proceeding, the prosecution's case against the defendant is presented by a city attorney, district attorney, or state's attorney, who is called the **prosecutor.** The defense attorney is a private attorney hired by the defendant. If the defendant can't afford an attorney, the judge will appoint an attorney to handle the defendant's case.

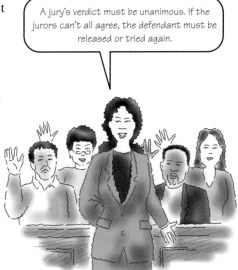

A jury's verdict must be unanimous. If the jurors can't all agree, the defendant must be released or tried again.

The Judge and the Jury

The judge conducts the trial and decides controversies over points of law and the introduction of evidence. The jury is a group of citizens from the community chosen to listen to the evidence presented and to decide the defendant's guilt or innocence. In a criminal case, this decision is called the **verdict.** If there is no jury, the judge decides the verdict. Whether there's a jury or not, if the verdict is "guilty," the judge then decides the defendant's punishment.

CIVIL LAW

Civil law covers wrongful acts that are not crimes. Under civil law, such charges arise when one party (the plaintiff), claims to have been injured by the actions of another party (the defendant) and sues the accused party. The plaintiff and defendant in a lawsuit are usually either a person or a business. But the government also can be a party in a suit under some circumstances.

Most civil suits fall into one of three categories.

- *Family issues.* These often involve matters such as divorce, child support, or disputes over child custody.

- *Contract disputes.* These often involve charges that someone has broken a contractual agreement. You'll read more about contracts later in this chapter.

- *Torts.* **Torts** are wrongs committed against a person or property that don't involve violation of a contract. Torts can be intentional or unintentional. You'll read more about torts in Chapter 3. Because some intentional torts can also be crimes, we're going to discuss them briefly now.

Intentional Torts

Intentional torts involve deliberate misconduct. Two common intentional torts are slander and libel.

- **Slander** is speaking lies about another person that harm the person's reputation or employment.
- **Libel** is damaging a person's reputation in writing.

For example, if you tell your coworkers that you've heard one of the nurses is an alcoholic—even though you don't know for sure that it's true—then you've slandered her. If you include this information in an e-mail to one of your coworkers, then you're guilty of libel. In either case, the nurse can sue you for your actions.

Here are some other intentional torts that might occur in a medical office. These torts can result in criminal charges in addition to a lawsuit:

- assault
- battery
- false imprisonment
- fraud

Assault

Assault is threatening a person or acting in a way that causes the person to fear harm. For example, suppose you're trying to examine a squirming child. If you threaten to strike the child if he doesn't remain still, you've just committed assault.

Battery

Battery is unlawful touching, whether or not the touching causes bodily harm. To avoid the tort of battery, you should never touch a patient without his consent. This doesn't necessarily mean that you have to ask permission, however. For example, if you're preparing to give a patient a flu shot and he rolls up his sleeve, he has indirectly given his consent. Or if you tell a patient that you're about to take her blood pressure and she doesn't object, this is also considered a form of consent.

False Imprisonment

Keeping a person against his will is false imprisonment. For example, suppose a patient who's waiting to see the physician decides he's waited long enough and is going to leave. If you tell him that he can't leave until he's paid for an office visit, this can be viewed as false imprisonment.

Fraud

Fraud is any dishonest practice that's intended to deceive another person. In a medical setting, convincing a patient to accept treatment by promising her a cure, when the treatment has no reasonable chance of curing her, would be one example of fraud.

Civil Trials

Most of the actions you just read about are crimes as well as torts. This means a person accused of doing them could be tried in criminal court in addition to being sued in civil court.

Civil cases are like criminal cases in many ways. But some important differences do exist.

- In a civil case, both parties are likely to be persons or businesses—for example, *Smith v. Jones* or *Taylor v. Acme Medical Clinic*. As you've already read, in a criminal case one party (the plaintiff) is *always* the government or "The People."

- The jury's decision does not have to be unanimous in a civil trial. If more than one-half of the jurors agree, a verdict has been reached. Also, the judge or jury in a civil case does not reach a "guilty" or "not guilty" verdict. Instead, the verdict is a finding in favor of the plaintiff or the defendant.

Accurate and thorough documentation is the best defense against lawsuits. If a conversation or treatment is not documented, it didn't happen.

If a case is decided in the plaintiff's favor, the jury (or judge, if there's no jury) also decides how much money the defendant must pay. Civil cases don't involve jail sentences; instead, the defendant must compensate the plaintiff for the harm he caused. This sum of money is called **compensatory damages.**

In some cases, a judge or jury may award a plaintiff money beyond the value of the harm done. This additional award is called **punitive damages.** Its purpose is to punish the defendant for especially bad behavior.

Defenses Against Torts

Of course, one response to charges of wrongdoing is to deny that it ever took place. In such situations, the best defense may be the patient's chart or medical record. That's one reason why it's important that all contact with a patient be accurately recorded in her chart. You'll read more about this subject in Chapter 7.

Other defenses in civil suits include the following.

- *Statute of limitations.* This is a legal time limit that exists for filing a lawsuit.
- *Respondeat superior.* This is a common law principle that employers are responsible for the actions of their employees.
- *Assumption of risk.* This is the principle that medical care involves risks that patients assume when they choose to seek treatment. Since this defense usually doesn't apply to intentional torts, it will be discussed in Chapter 4.

Statute of Limitations

Every state limits the length of time a patient has to file a suit against a health care provider. This time limit is called the **statute of limitations.** After that time, the person loses the right to sue.

Generally, the statute of limitations expires one to three years after the alleged tort took place. However, statutes of limitations vary from state to state. For example, in some states, the statute of limitations might be as long as eight years. Other variations occur because several states measure the time from the date that the patient *discovers* or *should have discovered* that wrongdoing may have occurred.

State laws also vary when the victim of an alleged tort is a minor. In such cases, the statute of limitations might not even begin until the patient becomes an adult. Then it might extend two or three years from that point. Some states also allow for longer statutes of limitations if the wrongdoing may have caused a patient's death.

To find the statute of limitations for your own state, contact the state board of medical examiners. The board's legal department should be able to provide you with information about the statute of limitations for your state and answer any questions you may have.

Respondeat Superior

Respondeat superior is a legal principle that is also known as the law of agency. It's a Latin term that means "let the master answer." This legal principle makes employers responsible for the actions of their employees. It's not a defense for your employer, but it can be an important protection for you if you're ever accused of a tort.

For example, imagine the physician you work for has asked you to administer an injection. You gather all your equipment, ensure that the five rights of administering an injection have been followed, and maintain aseptic technique. However, when

Legal Brief

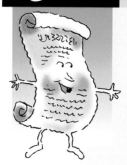

LET'S BE CIVIL HERE

> A contract is more than just an agreement. Certain conditions must be met for a contract to be legally binding.

Respondeat superior applies only to civil law. If an employee commits a crime, he can be arrested, brought to trial, and punished. The employer shares no responsibility for the crime unless the employer ordered, encouraged, or knowingly allowed the employee to commit it.

On the other hand, the statute of limitations applies to most crimes, as well as to charges of civil wrongdoing. This means that a person can't be charged with a crime after a set length of time has passed. Some crimes, such as murder, have no statute of limitations, however. Even if it takes 30 years to find a murder suspect, that person can still be charged with the crime.

you inject the needle into the patient, you inadvertently hit a nerve. The patient suffers nerve damage and sues. Under *respondeat superior,* even though the physician was not the person who administered the injection, she is ultimately responsible for your actions.

Keep in mind that *respondeat superior* is not always applicable. In a medical setting, your employer is responsible for your actions only when those actions are within your scope of practice. Your scope of practice is the range of tasks you're trained to perform. (You'll read more about this subject in Chapter 3.)

You should always be on guard against acting outside your scope of practice. If you do, your employer generally won't be legally responsible for your actions. If the result is a tort, you could be personally sued, and *respondeat superior* wouldn't protect you.

Contracts

A **contract** is a voluntary agreement between two parties from which each party benefits. If the agreement is spoken or put into writing, it's called an **expressed contract.** Contracts also can result from the behavior or actions of each party. This type of agreement is called an **implied contract.**

Whether a contract is expressed or implied, three conditions must exist to make it legally binding on each party.

- *Offer and acceptance.* One party makes an offer, and the other party accepts it. For example, a physician offers medical services by opening an office. Patients accept this offer by scheduling appointments.

- *Consideration.* Each party must exchange something of value with the other. The physician's consideration is the service she provides to the patient. The patient's consideration is payment of the physician's fee. Once each party has provided its consideration, the contract is complete.

- *Competence.* Each party must be able to understand the terms and conditions of the agreement. For example, a mentally incompetent person can't enter into a contract. Nor can a minor—which usually means anyone under age 18. That's why the consent of a parent or legal guardian is generally needed before treating a minor.

> A patient who's received a drug that interferes with judgment can't make a contract. Get consent for treatment before the patient is medicated.

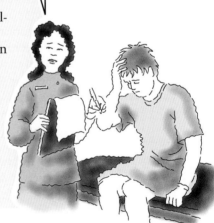

TREATING CHILDREN

About half of the states now consider children to be legal adults at age 14 when medical care is involved. Treating children under age 7 still requires the consent of a parent or legal guardian. For children between the ages of 7 and 14, the health care provider will determine on a case-by-case basis what the child's level of understanding and comprehension is and decide if the child is able to consent to her own treatment for conditions such as STDs or pregnancy.

EXPRESSED CONTRACTS

Some contracts a medical office makes must be in writing in order to be enforceable. These include third-party contracts and credit agreements. Usually, such contracts involve the payment of fees.

Third-Party Contracts

Suppose a man becomes ill but can't afford to see a physician. His adult daughter makes an appointment for him to see her physician. She tells the medical assistant that she'll pay the bill for her father's care. By making this promise, the daughter has entered into an expressed contract with the office.

This is not a typical expressed contract, however. It's different because the party who's receiving the physician's consideration (the patient) is not the one providing the return consideration (the daughter). A third party, who is receiving nothing of value from the physician, is completing the exchange. This type of contract is called a third-party contract, or a third-party payer contract.

Under common law, third-party contracts must be in writing to be legally binding. This means that unless the daughter signs a written contract to pay her father's bill, the office can't sue her if she later refuses to pay. The office can sue the father to collect its fees, but he may not have the means to pay.

Insurance policies are another type of third-party payer contract. Whether a third-party payer is involved or not, most offices require patients to sign written agreements to pay any charges not paid by insurance. These agreements should be signed before treatment begins.

Credit Agreements

Another financial matter that can involve a written contract is an agreement with a patient to pay his bill over time. Federal law requires written contracts for credit arrangements under the following four conditions.

1. The credit is offered to the consumer of the goods or services.
2. The business offers credit on a regular basis.

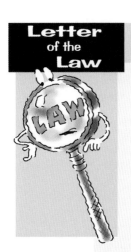

Letter of the Law

THE CONSUMER PROTECTION ACT

The Consumer Protection Act of 1968 governs payment arrangements that health care providers may make with patients to pay their bills. It requires that the contracts signed by patients must contain the following information:

- total amount for which the patient is responsible
- amount of any down payment the patient has made
- amount of each installment and when it is due
- date of the final payment
- amount of interest, if any, the office is charging the patient

3. Interest will be charged, or the bill will be paid in more than four installments.

4. The credit extended is for personal or family use.

The patient must be given a copy of the signed credit contract. A second copy should be placed in the patient's billing records.

IMPLIED CONTRACTS

Implied contracts are contracts in which agreement between the parties is not shown by words, but by action, lack of action, or silence. Implied contracts are very common in a medical office. Here's a typical example: A patient describes her symptoms to the physician. The physician examines the patient, writes her a prescription, and tells her to schedule a follow-up appointment.

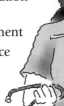

Never promise a patient that a treatment will make him better. If it fails to do so, the patient could sue for breach of contract.

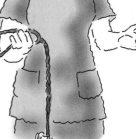

A contract has been made in this example, even though it was never directly stated. Both parties must now follow through on their implied agreement. The patient is responsible for:

- filling the prescription and taking the medication as instructed
- making and keeping the follow-up appointment
- paying the bill if it is not covered by insurance

The physician has obligations, too. He must:

- be willing to see the patient again
- continue to treat her if her condition persists

If either party fails to do these things, the contract has been broken. This is known as **breach of contract.** Breach of contract occurs when either party fails to live up to the terms of the agreement.

TERMINATION

The contract usually ends when the patient's treatment is complete and the physician has been paid. However, sometimes issues arise that cause a contract to end before both parties have fulfilled their obligations.

The patient has the right to terminate the contract at any time. Under certain circumstances, the physician also has a right to end a contract early. The physician may want to end the physician-patient relationship for personal reasons. More often, however, breach of contract is the reason for early termination.

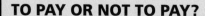

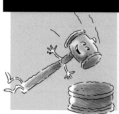

What's the Verdict? | **TO PAY OR NOT TO PAY?**

A man sees a physician seeking treatment for a sore throat and fatigue. After examining the patient's throat and lymph nodes, the physician tells the patient, "I'd like to take some blood and test for mononucleosis." He then takes the patient to a different room to have the medical assistant take a blood sample. The medical assistant explains the procedure and asks the patient to roll up his sleeve. She draws the blood with no complications and sends the specimen to the lab.

When the patient gets the bill for the office visit, it includes an additional fee of $35 for venipuncture. Since the patient never signed a consent form for this procedure, he believes that he should not have to pay this charge. Should he have to pay?

The Verdict: The patient must pay for the venipuncture. He did not object when the medical assistant told him what was going to happen and he rolled up his sleeve to allow the medical assistant to perform the task. In doing this, the patient gave his implied consent to the procedure. An implied contract was created. The medical assistant did her part by performing the procedure. The patient must now fulfill his part of the contract by paying the charge for it.

Breach of Contract

A physician may terminate a contract with a patient in the following situations, each of which involves breach of contract.

- The patient does not keep appointments.
- The patient does not follow the physician's instructions.
- The patient fails to pay his bill.

Abandonment

If the physician wishes to terminate the contract and the patient still seeks treatment, the physician must follow specific legal procedures to end the physician-patient relationship. If the physician doesn't terminate the contract properly, the patient can sue for **abandonment.**

Abandonment occurs when the physician ends the relationship without proper notice while the patient still needs treatment.

By the Book   TERMINATING A CONTRACT

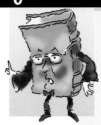

To end the contract with a patient and avoid a charge of abandonment, the office must send the patient a letter. As a medical assistant, you may be responsible for preparing this letter. Here's what it must contain:

- a statement that the physician intends to end the relationship
- the reasons for this action
- a termination date that is at least 30 days from the date on the letter
- a statement that the patient's medical records will be transferred to another office at the patient's request
- a recommendation urging the patient to seek any additional medical care that may be required

The termination letter must be sent by certified mail with a return receipt requested. Place a copy of the letter and the returned receipt in the patient's record.

> Send all termination letters by certified mail. And be sure to request a return receipt.

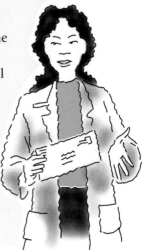

Here are some other situations that also can be considered abandonment.

- The physician doesn't see the patient as often as the patient's condition requires.
- The physician incorrectly tells the patient that no more treatment is needed.
- The physician does not arrange for another physician to care for the patient when the physician must be away.

We're Being Sued!

Only about one of every ten lawsuits brought by patients against health care providers actually ends up in court. If the patient's case is very weak, the judge may dismiss it before the trial even begins. Other suits are settled out of court by agreement between the plaintiff, the defendant, and the defendant's liability insurance company. If there's a settlement, the defendant may agree to pay the plaintiff a certain amount of money to avoid going to trial.

Settlements also may be reached at any time once the trial is under way—until the jury actually reaches a verdict. In fact, only about one in a hundred lawsuits that are filed actually reach a final decision by a judge or a jury.

But no matter how the case ends, lawsuits can cause great stress in a medical office. Health care providers can become concerned for their jobs, their reputations, and their ability to practice their profession. Staff members may have extra demands on their time as the office prepares to defend against the suit.

There's a popular saying in health care, "The rude get sued!"

Here's what to expect from the time a suit is filed to its possible conclusion in court.

THE COMPLAINT

If a patient suspects that something went wrong with her treatment, she may first seek information from the medical office. In many cases, she will view the physician as unapproachable and direct her questions to the medical assistant. This creates a delicate situation, which must be handled with both caution and tact. On one hand, you should not provide any information without the physician's approval. On the other hand, you must try to avoid angering the patient.

If the patient does not get satisfactory answers at the medical office, her next step probably will be to consult an attorney. The attorney will request a copy of the patient's medical records and may also have another physician examine the patient. If the attorney thinks the patient has a case, he'll probably contact the medical office, or its attorney, about a settlement.

If settlement negotiations fail, the attorney's next step will be to file a written charge of wrongdoing, called a **complaint,** with the court. The complaint will explain in detail the torts or other violations of civil law the attorney believes have occurred. The court then serves the medical office with a copy of the complaint. At this point, the patient becomes the plaintiff, and the office becomes the defendant. Office employees who were involved in the patient's care probably will be named as defendants, too.

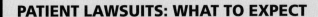

Exhibits

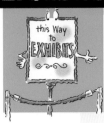

PATIENT LAWSUITS: WHAT TO EXPECT

The first action in a patient lawsuit starts when the patient files a complaint. The following steps describe what you can expect:

1. If the patient feels that there was a problem with his treatment, the first thing he will do is discuss his concerns with the medical office staff. If he finds the answers acceptable and fair, he might not take legal action. If he still feels there was wrongdoing, he will be on his way to a lawsuit.

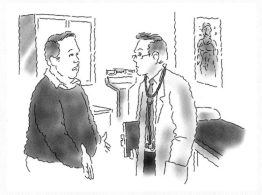

2. Next, the patient will contact an attorney to discuss his problem. The attorney will request the patient's medical records from the medical office and may have her new client get a second opinion.

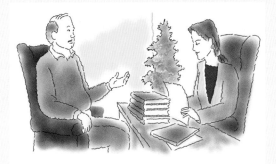

3. If the attorney finds that the patient has a case, she'll contact the medical office or its legal representation to see about a settlement.

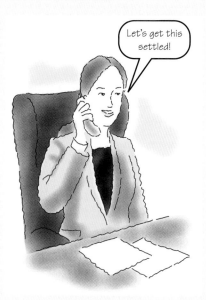

4. If the attorney and medical office can't reach a settlement, the attorney will file the complaint with the court. The court in turn serves the medical office with a copy of this complaint. The legal battle in court is officially underway.

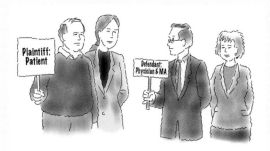

DISCOVERY

Discovery is a legal process to uncover facts about the situation before the trial begins. Both sides conduct discovery. It can include the following actions.

- **Subpoenas** are orders issued by the court to obtain evidence. The term subpoena is often used to refer to an order requiring you to provide spoken testimony in court as evidence in a trial. However, you may also encounter another form of subpoena in the medical office. *Subpoena duces tecum* is an order requiring you or your employer to provide evidence in the form of documents to the court.

- **Interrogatories** are written questions about the case that each side submits to the other. These questions must be answered truthfully and in writing.

- **Depositions** are oral answers that the parties to the case and witnesses provide to questions by each side's attorney before the trial begins. They are made under oath and may be used as evidence at trial.

- **Motions** are requests to the judge on which he must rule. One motion the defense usually makes is that the case be **dismissed**, or thrown out of court. The judge generally does not rule on this motion until each side has been heard at the pretrial conference.

Negotiations to settle the case out of court often continue during the discovery phase and the pretrial conference.

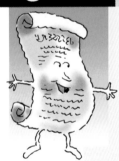

Legal Brief   COLLECTING EVIDENCE

As a medical assistant, it may be your job to gather records subpoenaed in a lawsuit. Here are some guidelines to follow.

- Unless instructed otherwise by your employer, do not provide records unless they've been subpoenaed.
- Provide only the exact records listed on the subpoena— nothing more or less.
- Unless the subpoena asks for original records, provide only photocopies. Again, copy only what has been asked for.
- If the subpoena requires original records, make a copy of them to replace the originals in the office files.

THE PRETRIAL CONFERENCE

The pretrial conference is the first meeting of the plaintiff and the defendant in court. Its main purpose is to determine if the case for wrongdoing is strong enough to proceed to trial. After hearing arguments from both sides, the judge may rule on the defense's motion to dismiss the case. If the motion is granted, the case ends. If the case is not dismissed, either side may present a motion for a jury trial.

THE TRIAL

If the case is not settled or dismissed, it goes to trial. During the trial, each side produces evidence and witnesses that present the facts of the case as that side sees them. In a jury trial, 6 to 12 citizens from the community decide whose "facts" are correct and make a decision in favor of the plaintiff or the defendant. In a bench trial, the judge does this job. The judge also decides any points of law that arise during the trial.

Opening Arguments

The trial begins with opening arguments. They consist of a short speech by each side's attorney and state what each attorney intends to prove during the trial.

The Plaintiff's Case

The plaintiff's attorney presents evidence and calls witnesses first. Each witness swears to tell the truth and then, under questioning by the attorney, tells what he knows about the situation that caused the suit. Then the witness can be cross-examined by the defense attorney. The defense attorney asks questions of the witness that are designed to weaken the witness's testimony and the plaintiff's case.

The Defendant's Case

After the plaintiff's case has been presented, it's the defendant's turn. Witnesses and evidence for the defendant's version of events are introduced. Like the plaintiff's witnesses, some defense witnesses may be **expert witnesses.** These are witnesses with special professional or technical knowledge that can help shed light on the facts of the case. The defendant may be called as a witness, but he can't be required to testify.

After the defense witnesses have been cross-examined by the plaintiff's attorney, each side "rests," or ends its case.

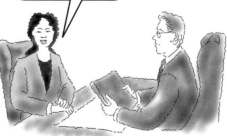

If you're called as a witness in a lawsuit, your employer's attorney will help you prepare your testimony.

By the Book   TIPS FOR TESTIFYING

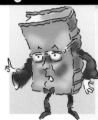

If you're asked to testify as a witness in a lawsuit, here are some points to remember.

- *Require a subpoena.* It's best not to volunteer to be a witness, especially if you'll be testifying against an employer or coworker. But if you're subpoenaed, you have to appear whether you want to testify or not.

- *Be truthful.* You'll be testifying under oath. This means that if you lie, you'll be committing perjury, which is a crime. Also remember that if you gave a deposition before the trial began, your answers there will be compared to your answers in court. Major differences can make your testimony less believable.

- *Be professional.* The image you present contributes to whether your statements are considered believable. Be dignified and remain calm and serious at all times.

- *Answer the question.* But do not give any information that was not asked for. Unless you're asked for your opinion, give only the facts. If you don't know something, say so.

- *Cooperate with your side's attorney.* If your attorney objects to a question from the other side's attorney, don't answer the question unless the judge tells you to do so.

- *Pay attention.* It's important to pay attention, especially when you're being cross-examined. The opposing attorney will be trying to get you to say things that will weaken your side's case. Think before you speak. If you get tired and your mind starts to wander, ask the judge for a **recess.** This is a short break in the trial.

Closing Arguments and Jury Instructions

The trial ends with the attorneys for each side summarizing the case they presented. Next, in a jury trial, the judge instructs the jury about the law as it applies to the case. Then the jury goes to another room so it can consider the evidence that's been presented and come to a decision about the case. As you read earlier in this chapter, if the jury decides the case for the plaintiff, the jury also must decide how much to award in damages.

If the judge or jury finds for the defendant, the case is over. The plaintiff can't sue the defendant again for the same issue. But either side can appeal the decision to a higher court.

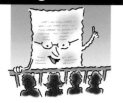

Closing Statements

- Laws come from three sources: legislative, executive, and judicial branches.
- The three different types of law are statutory, administrative, and case law.
- Criminal law involves felonies and misdemeanors.
- In criminal cases, the government (the plaintiff or prosecution) charges a defendant with breaking a federal, state, or local law. A judge or jury must decide the case by declaring the accused "guilty" or "not guilty."
- Civil law covers wrongful acts that aren't crimes, including family issues, contract disputes, and torts.
- Civil suits come about when one party (the plaintiff) claims to be injured by the actions of another party (the defendant) and sues the accused party. A judge or jury then finds in favor of the plaintiff or defendant and awards damages, if applicable.
- In the medical office, *respondeat superior* means your employer is responsible for your actions when you act within your scope of practice.
- For a contract to be valid, three things must be present: offer and acceptance, consideration, and competence.
- Contracts may be expressed in writing or implied through action or lack of action.
- When terminating a contract, the physician must notify the patient by letter, allowing the patient 30 days to choose another physician. The letter should state the reason for termination, make the patient's records available for transfer to another physician, and recommend further treatments and care, if necessary.
- The litigation process involves a complaint, discovery, a pretrial conference, and a trial.
- In a lawsuit, a plaintiff first files a complaint. Then, the plaintiff and defendant's attorneys conduct discovery. A judge presides over the pretrial conference; during the trial, a judge or jury decides the case.

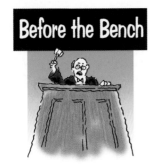

Before the Bench

Answer the following multiple-choice questions.

1. The main source of criminal law is:
   a. the court system.
   b. the legislative branch of government.
   c. executive agencies.
   d. state governments.

2. Who is always the plaintiff in a criminal case?
   a. the government
   b. the person accused of a crime
   c. the judge
   d. the person who has been harmed

3. What legal principle protects a medical assistant who behaves correctly but is sued?
   a. statute of limitations
   b. *stare decisis*
   c. *respondeat superior*
   d. common law

4. An action that harms a person or property but is not a crime is called:
   a. a misdemeanor.
   b. fraud.
   c. abuse.
   d. a tort.

5. The two parties in a lawsuit can agree to settle the dispute out of court until:
   a. a complaint is filed with the court.
   b. the pretrial conference is held.
   c. the defense rests its case in the trial.
   d. the jury reaches a verdict.

6. An implied contract can exist if two parties:
   a. sign a document in which each promises do something.
   b. both act in a way that indicates they agree to something.
   c. state their agreement in front of witnesses.
   d. each perform a service for the other for free.

7. Which of the following is *not* considered a breach of contract?
   a. The patient consistently fails to keep his appointments with the physician.
   b. The physician refuses to prescribe a certain drug the patient wants to take.
   c. The physician sends the patient a letter terminating the physician-patient relationship.
   d. The patient refuses to take the medicine the physician has prescribed.

8. Which behavior by a medical assistant could cause her employer to be sued for breach of contract?
   a. promising a patient that the treatment he has just received will make him better
   b. filing a claim with an insurance company for a service the physician did not perform
   c. lying on the witness stand in a patient's lawsuit against the employer
   d. calling a patient to reschedule an appointment because the physician is ill

9. What is another name for civil law?
   a. common law
   b. private law
   c. federal law
   d. administrative law

10. When is the *only* time you should provide someone with the original of a patient's medical record?
    a. if the patient has signed a release of medical records
    b. if the patient's attorney asks for it
    c. if photocopies of the records are not readable
    d. if the original record is subpoenaed

Chapter 3

MEDICAL PRACTICE AND THE LAW

Chapter Checklist

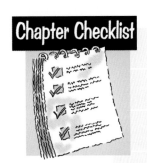

- Describe the medical assistant's scope of practice and explain where the assistant should go if he or she has questions

- Explain standard of care as it relates to physicians and medical assistants

- Explain the difference between intentional and unintentional torts

- Define what a tortfeasor is

- Define and explain the difference between malfeasance, misfeasance, and nonfeasance

- Identify the four Ds of negligence

Chapter Competencies

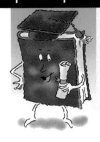

- Perform within legal and ethical boundaries (CAAHEP 3.c.2.b.)

- Conduct work within scope of education, training, and ability (ABHES 1.i.)

- Identify and respond to issues of confidentiality (CAAHEP 3.c.2.a.)

- Maintain confidentiality at all times (ABHES 1.b.)

There are a great many ways that health care providers can get into trouble for things they might do—or fail to do—in the medical office. This chapter will provide you with some basic guidelines for behaving lawfully and ethically in your work as a medical assistant. It will also alert you to the kinds of behaviors you should avoid if you want your career in medical assisting to be a pleasant and successful one.

The Scoop on Scope of Practice

Every employee in a medical office must be careful to work within his scope of practice. A **scope of practice** is the range of activities that a health care worker is qualified to perform. In most cases, being "qualified" depends on the employee's level of education and training. For some medical professionals, such as physicians and nurses, scope of practice is determined by the laws governing the license they hold.

For medical assistants, scope of practice is less clear for a number of reasons.

- No state offers licenses to medical assistants.
- Training for medical assistants varies. Fewer medical assistants are receiving on-the-job training than in the past. Today, physicians are more likely to hire medical assistants trained in a formal environment because they don't have enough time for training on the job. Formal training can range from a few months of vocational school to two-year degree programs at community colleges.

However, despite these obstacles, a general scope of practice for medical assistants does exist.

THE PRACTICE OF MEDICAL ASSISTING

Most states allow medical assistants to perform certain duties under the supervision of a licensed practitioner, such as a physician or podiatrist. In fact, more than half the states allow a physician to assign basic clinical tasks to a medical assistant under the following conditions:

- the state's medical practice and nursing practice laws don't limit the task to physicians or nurses
- the medical assistant has the training to carry out the task safely
- the medical assistant carries out the task under the physician's supervision

- the physician takes responsibility for the medical assistant's actions

A few states have laws that recognize the profession of medical assisting. Some of them even provide a scope of practice for medical assistants. South Dakota's law is a good example of a general guide. On the other hand, Arizona relies largely on the clinical and administrative competencies for medical assistants established by the Commission on Accreditation of Allied Health Education Programs (CAAHEP). These competencies are the skills you must master if you want to become a Certified Medical Assistant (CMA) by the American Association of Medical Assistants (AAMA) or a Registered Medical Assistant (RMA) by the American Medical Technologists (AMT).

> This book and the others in this series are designed to help you become a Certified Medical Assistant (CMA) or a Registered Medical Assistant (RMA).

THE AAMA AND SCOPE OF PRACTICE

In 2002, the AAMA surveyed more than 15,000 medical assistants across the United States to find out what they actually were doing on the job. Responses showed that medical assistants perform a wide variety of duties. Top tasks included:

- assisting in clinical and patient care procedures, including intravenous procedures
- providing patient education
- performing medical coding and billing
- handling medical records
- performing management and supervisory tasks

Some medical assistants have administrative as well as clinical duties, and many are cross-trained to work in both areas. Common administrative tasks include:

- answering phones and scheduling appointments
- greeting patients
- arranging for hospital admissions and lab services
- updating and filing patient medical records
- coding and filling out insurance claim forms
- handling correspondence, billing, and bookkeeping

As you've already read, your clinical duties as a medical assistant can depend on the laws of the state where you work. They also can depend on the size and specialty of your medical office. But the AAMA has compiled a list of common clinical tasks for medical assistants. These tasks include:

- taking medical histories
- explaining treatment procedures to patients
- preparing patients for examination
- assisting the physician during the examination
- collecting and preparing laboratory specimens
- performing basic laboratory tests
- instructing patients about medications and special diets
- preparing and giving medications as directed by the physician
- authorizing prescription refills as directed
- performing venipuncture
- taking ECGs
- removing sutures and changing dressings

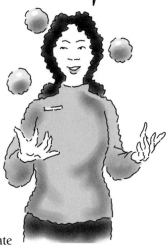

Multiskilled medical assistants trained in both administrative and clinical skills are more valuable to the practice!

SCOPE OF PRACTICE DOS AND DON'TS

It's important for you to be aware of any limits your state puts on the activities of medical assistants—especially in the clinical area. For example, in some states, medical assistants may initiate and administer IVs. However, as you'll read in the *Legal Brief* on the next page, this is not permitted in other states.

It's the physician's responsibility to know what medical assistants can and can't do—either as set by state law or by a medical assistant's training and experience. A physician must not assign you activities that are beyond your scope of practice. Nor can the physician assign you tasks that are clearly not permitted by your state's laws. It's equally important that you don't perform them on your own. Exceeding your scope of practice—whether by the physician's order or on your own—is unethical as well as illegal. You're only covered under your physician's malpractice insurance if you're acting within your scope of practice. So, not only is exceeding your scope of practice poor customer service to patients, but it could also get both you and your employer sued!

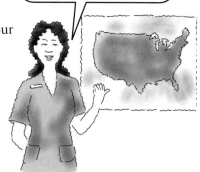

Remember that laws regarding tasks that you can and can't perform vary from state to state. Check with your instructor or supervisor to find out which tasks you're permitted to complete in your state.

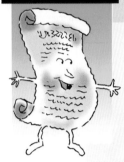

Legal Brief   LIMITS ON MEDICAL ASSISTANTS' SCOPE OF PRACTICE

As you've already read, medical assistants' scope of practice varies from state to state. Here are some tasks that medical assistants *cannot* perform in most states:

- independently diagnose symptoms, interpret test results, or treat patients

- advise patients about their condition or treatment

- independently write or refill prescriptions or give out medication samples

- flush, or discontinue IVs or inject medications into **veins** (vessels that carry blood from other parts of the body to the heart)

- insert urinary **catheters** (tubes used to drain fluid from the body) or perform punctures of **arteries** (vessels that carry blood from the heart to other parts of the body)

- perform tests that involve penetration of human tissues, except for skin tests and drawing blood from veins, where permitted by law

- administer **anesthetics** (substances that make the body unable, or less able, to feel pain), except for anesthetic skin creams

- operate laser equipment, practice physical therapy, or place splints on injured limbs

> If you don't feel qualified to perform a task, speak up! It's your responsibility to let the physician know.

By the Book   STAYING WITHIN YOUR SCOPE OF PRACTICE

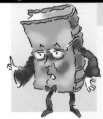

It's your responsibility to question any task that you don't feel comfortable doing. Remember that the physician may not be aware of your personal level of training, experience, or level of confidence when assigning a task to you. It's your responsibility to inform the physician if you feel uncomfortable performing a particular task.

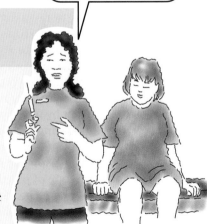

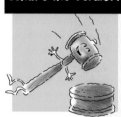

What's the Verdict? **AM I GOING TO DIE?**

Charles is a medical assistant in an oncologist's office. (An ***oncologist*** *is a physician who specializes in treating cancer.) A patient was visibly upset after her treatment as she and Charles arranged an appointment for her next visit. "I'm going to die, aren't I?" she blurted out, as tears welled up in her eyes. Charles knew that patients with her type of cancer have a high cure rate. "Don't worry," he told her. "You're going to be just fine." The comforted patient thanked him and left the office greatly relieved. Did Charles provide an acceptable standard of care in this situation?*

The Verdict: No. Charles acted honestly and openly, but he exceeded his scope of practice by advising the patient about her condition. As a medical assistant, he does not have the education to make such a judgment. Also, while Charles may have a basic knowledge of cancer, he does not have the training to know how other health factors might affect her condition and outcome. Not only has Charles almost promised a cure, he may actually have given the patient false hope. The best response would be to show empathy and refer the patient's question to the nurse or physician.

Living Up to Standards

So, you understand the importance of working within your scope of practice. But your legal and ethical responsibilities as a medical assistant don't end there. You must also provide an acceptable standard of care. **Standard of care** is the level of performance that's expected of a health care worker in carrying out assigned duties.

Like scope of practice, standard of care is closely linked to education and training. For example, physicians are held to a higher standard of care than are medical assistants. That's because physicians have more training than medical assistants do.

Unlike your scope of practice, your standard of care as a medical assistant does not depend on your *own* skills and training. That's because the standard of care for each medical profession is set by the knowledge that's typical for workers in that profession. No matter what your own background is, the standard of care expected from you depends on what's reasonable to expect from the average medical assistant. This is called the **reasonable person standard.**

You'll read more about the reasonable person standard later in the chapter. It's an important part of standard of care. Both standard of care and scope of practice are important in avoiding the legal problems you'll read about later in this chapter.

DUTY OF CARE

Duty of care is another important part of standard of care. **Duty of care** is the legal obligation, or duty, a health care worker has to patients and sometimes to nonpatients as well.

For example, as you learned in previous chapters, you must keep a patient's health information private and confidential. If you don't, you've breached your duty of care to the patient and have therefore not provided the proper standard of care. (A **breach** is a failure to do what's required.) You'll read more about both topics—breach of duty and confidentiality—later in this chapter.

DUTY OF CARE TO COWORKERS

Here's an example of duty of care to nonpatients. Your office has special containers for disposal of hazardous materials such as used needles. You owe a duty of care to your coworkers to use these containers instead of tossing needles into the regular trash, where the used needles could injure other employees.

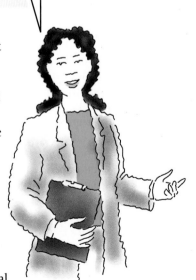

Physicians do sometimes make mistakes. As a medical assistant, it's one of your responsibilities to serve as a second set of eyes and ears to help keep these mistakes from causing harm.

The Duty of Obedience

The duty to follow orders is a duty of care that you owe both to your employer and to your patients. It includes the duty to:

- interpret the physician's instructions and carry them out
- ask for clarification if the instructions are unclear or seem wrong
- immediately tell the physician *if* orders appear to be harmful or dangerous for the patient. You must *not* follow any orders that seem inappropriate.

The Duty of Truth

You read about honesty as an ethical require-ment in Chapter 1. But telling the truth is a legal

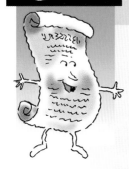

Legal Brief

DUTY OF CARE AND
RESPONDEAT SUPERIOR

As you learned in Chapter 2, *respondeat superior* is the legal principle that your employer is responsible for your actions if you're acting within your scope of practice. However, *respondeat superior* may not apply if by following the physician's orders you harm a patient, and then you don't let the physician know. Case law has established that failing to tell the physician breaches your duty of care to the patient. If you do not tell the physician, the physician can't correct the situation. For example, a medical assistant instructed to administer an intramuscular injection accidentally hits the sciatic nerve while administering the shot. If the medical assistant lets the patient leave and does not tell the physician, the patient may return to the office due to pain from the shot. In almost every case of this type, the courts have ruled that *both* the employer and the employee must pay damages to the patient.

duty, too. It means that health care professionals must deal honestly and openly with patients at all times. Patients have a right to know their past and current medical status. This includes being told when their diagnosis changes as test results and other information are analyzed. It also involves making sure patients understand the risks of any treatments they agree to have.

Although you must never lie to a patient, you must also be very careful to avoid exceeding your scope of practice when providing information to patients. If you have any concerns about information a patient is asking you to provide or explain, you should always refer the patient to the physician for an answer. It's better to err on the side of caution and not release the information than to release and hope that it turns out well.

THE REASONABLE PERSON STANDARD

Has a health care worker provided an acceptable standard of care to a patient? Has the worker met his duty of care to the patient? Both questions are central to knowing whether a patient who feels wronged has a legal case against the health care provider. One way such questions are answered in court is by applying the reasonable person standard.

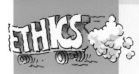

Ethics in Action HONESTY: AN ETHICAL DILEMMA

The duty to be honest and open can be complicated in some cases. Consider the following situations.

- Should a physician tell an older adult patient whose family is secretly arranging to place the patient in a nursing home?
- If a patient dies during a treatment, should a medical assistant mislead the patient's family when calling them to come to the office, especially knowing they'll be driving?
- Should a physician violate patient confidentiality and warn the police that a patient has threatened to kill her husband?

These kinds of situations are made even more difficult by the fact that there often isn't a clear "right" answer.

The reasonable person standard is a legal principle that every person has a duty to behave as a "reasonable person" would in the same circumstances. What's "reasonable" partly depends on the person involved. For example, a nurse who's treating victims at an accident scene would be held to a higher standard of reasonable behavior than a person with no medical training. The standard for the nurse would be the behavior that could reasonably be expected from a nurse in that situation. The question that is usually asked is, "What would someone with the same level of training have done in this situation?"

MEDICAL ASSISTANTS AND REASONABLE BEHAVIOR

Failing to meet the reasonable person standard—in your case, what's reasonable behavior for a medical assistant in a particular situation—could lead to charges of negligence. **Negligence** is the failure to act with proper or reasonable care.

Torts: No Harm, No Foul

As you learned in Chapter 2, torts are wrongful acts committed against a person or property. **Intentional torts** are deliberate acts that cause harm. For this reason, many intentional torts are also crimes. **Unintentional torts** are accidental rather than

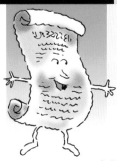

Legal Brief　DELAYED TORTS

Every treatment error in a medical office must be reported, even if it does not seem to have harmed the patient. That's because an error's harmful effects may not appear right away. If and when harmful effects do appear, that's the point at which the statute of limitations begins to run.

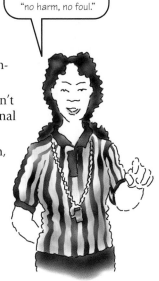

In the tort world, it's "no harm, no foul."

deliberate. In these cases, the **tortfeasor** (the person who commits the tort) does not mean to harm the person or property.

- Running someone down with your car is an intentional tort (and a crime).
- Hitting someone with your car because you weren't paying attention to your driving is an unintentional tort (and negligence).

In either case, a tort always involves some sort of harm, whether it's mental, emotional, or physical.

If you hit someone with your car because you aren't paying attention to your driving, you're negligent because a reasonable person would be paying attention. Your inattentive behavior does not meet the reasonable person standard and makes you guilty of the tort of negligence.

Tort cases are tried in civil courts, and the injured person may recover money damages from the tortfeasor. Intentional torts can also be tried as crimes in criminal courts. The tortfeasor becomes the defendant and can be jailed or fined if he is found guilty. A criminal court can't award damages to the injured party, however. To collect damages, the injured party must sue the tortfeasor in a separate action in civil court.

NEGLIGENCE AND MALPRACTICE

As you just learned, negligence results from failing to act with reasonable care, causing harm to another person. Negligence can occur in either of two ways:

- by doing something that a reasonable person would *not* do
- by *not* doing something that a reasonable person *would* do

When a professional person is negligent in his or her duties, it's known as **malpractice.** Negligence by a medical professional is called medical malpractice. This separate category for negligence by professionals is based on the principle that their level of knowledge gives them a greater duty of care than the reasonable person standard requires.

Like ordinary negligence, harm or injury must result for malpractice to occur. Accusations of malpractice are the most common reason for lawsuits against health care professionals. There are three types of malpractice claims:

- malfeasance—taking an improper action
- misfeasance—taking a proper action but in an improper way
- nonfeasance—not taking a necessary action

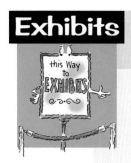

Exhibits

MALFEASANCE, MISFEASANCE, AND NONFEASANCE

Malfeasance is the performance of a wrong and unlawful act. For example, a medical assistant who tells a patient to treat her symptoms by taking an aspirin is committing an act of malfeasance because only a physician can prescribe treatments.

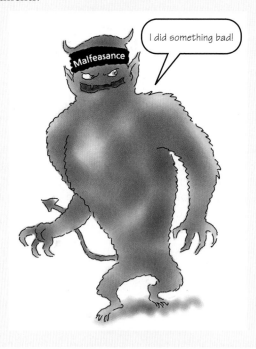

Misfeasance is the performance of a lawful act in an improper manner. For example, a medical assistant fails to use a sterile bandage when dressing a patient's wound, resulting in an infection for the patient.

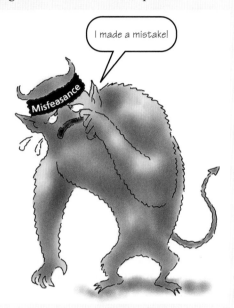

Nonfeasance is the failure to perform a necessary act. For example, a patient stops breathing in the waiting room, and the medical assistant, who is trained in CPR, does not perform CPR on the patient.

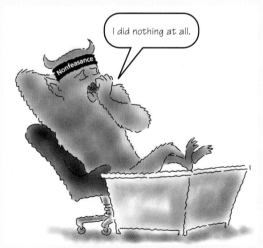

THE FOUR Ds OF NEGLIGENCE

For a health care provider to be sued for malpractice successfully, the plaintiff (the accuser) usually must prove four things. They are sometimes called the "four Ds of negligence":

- *Duty*—the responsibility to provide a reasonable standard of care to the patient
- *Dereliction of duty*—not providing a reasonable standard of care to the patient
- *Direct or proximate cause*—the direct or indirect cause of a patient's injury
- *Damages*—the harm suffered by a patient

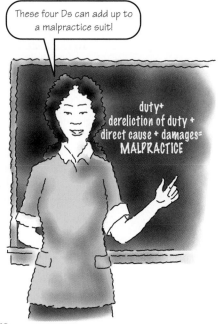

These four Ds can add up to a malpractice suit!

duty+
dereliction of duty +
direct cause + damages=
MALPRACTICE

Cause

To prove *direct cause*, there must be an unbroken chain of events that connect the improper action to the harm done. For example:

1. a child comes in sick.
2. the medical assistant administers an adult dosage of medication to the child.
3. the child dies as a result of the overmedication.

In this example, the medical assistant's failure to provide the proper dosage to the child was the direct cause of the patient's death.

However, it isn't always possible to prove direct cause. Suppose EMS had come, revived the patient, and taken her to the hospital, where she later died. Proving malpractice would require proving that the medical assistant's failure to administer the correct dosage was the *proximate cause* of the patient's death. That is, it must be proven that some intervening act—such as a medication error in the hospital—didn't cause the death instead.

Damages

Many kinds of damages can cause patients to seek financial compensation from the accused in a malpractice case. **Compensation** is something good that is given to reduce the bad effect

Legal Brief   *RES IPSA LOQUITUR*

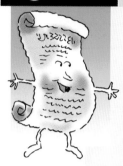

Sometimes a patient does not have to prove the four Ds to win a malpractice suit. In some cases the common law doctrine of *res ipsa loquitur* applies. (A **doctrine** is a principle of law.) *Res ipsa loquitur* is a Latin term that means "the thing speaks for itself." Operating on the wrong leg to fix a broken leg is a perfect example of when a patient would claim *res ipsa loquitur* in court. In an instance such as this, the surgeon's mistake would be so obvious that no more evidence is needed. For this reason, surgeons now verify the leg that needs the operation with the patient along with two or three other witnesses well before the surgery takes place. They then mark the correct leg to make sure no mistakes are made during surgery. These precautions help keep patients safer and also protect the surgeon from committing *res ipsa loquitur*.

Three conditions must exist for the doctrine of *res ipsa loquitur* to apply:

- The defendant had direct and complete control over the cause of the injury.
- The injury would not have occurred if the defendant had exercised reasonable care.
- The plaintiff (patient) did not in any way contribute to the cause of the injury.

When a plaintiff claims *res ipsa loquitur*, the burden of proof shifts to the defendant. The defendant must prove that negligence did *not* occur.

of some damage, loss, or injury. Some of the more common reasons for financial compensation in malpractice cases are:

- personal injury
- pain and suffering
- mental anguish
- loss of enjoyment of life
- permanent physical or mental disability
- loss of past and future income
- hospital and medical expenses

DAMAGES AND COMPENSATION

When malpractice causes a patient's death, a family member will often be the plaintiff in the lawsuit against the health care provider. This is called a wrongful death suit. In that case, the compensation the defendant must pay can be based on harm done to the plaintiff as well as to the patient. For example, the patient's spouse or parent (if the patient was a child) will likely have suffered mental anguish from the death. If the patient was employed, the spouse will have suffered loss of income, too. In fact, "loss of service" of spouse or child is a common cause for damage awards if malpractice kills a patient.

> Don't get confused! The term *damages* has two meanings in law—both the harm done and the money the defendant must pay.

Can You Keep a Secret?

One of the most important duties of care that you—and all health care professionals—owe to patients is the confidentiality of their personal information. Breaking patient confidentiality is a breach of professional ethics as well as a serious violation of federal law.

PATIENT PRIVACY AND HIPAA

The Health Insurance Portability and Accountability Act of 1996 (HIPAA) protects the privacy of a patient's personal and health information. This law has brought sweeping changes to the health care industry. Its original purpose was to:

- improve health benefits for workers who change jobs
- reduce costs by streamlining the health care system
- simplify the processing of health insurance claims

As medical offices and other health care providers increasingly used computers in the 1970s and 1980s for office tasks, lawmakers saw the need for new privacy legislation. Computers began replacing the old "hand" systems for:

- billing patients, recording payments, and keeping track of patients' accounts
- scheduling patients' appointments and storing their contact information, health insurance information, and other personal data

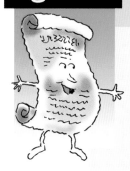

Legal Brief

THE PRICE FOR BREAKING CONFIDENTIALITY

If you fail to protect patient confidentiality, federal law prohibits the patient from suing for malpractice. However, the federal government can fine you or your employer up to $25,000 per offense. If your action was deliberate, you can also be required to pay criminal penalties of $50,000 to $250,000 and serve time in federal prison. As you can see, patient confidentiality is a big deal!

Except where its release is required or allowable by law, all information about a patient is confidential. You'll learn more about patient confidentiality—and when it does not apply—when you read Chapters 6 and 7. In general, however, here are some basic things you need to know on this subject to avoid allegations of breach of duty and malpractice.

- All of a patient's personal data are confidential, including name and address, phone number, employment information, and insurance information.

- All health information is confidential. This includes the patient's medical history, diagnosis, tests ordered, test results, treatments, medications administered in the office, and prescriptions.

- All written or oral communication between the patient and medical office employees is confidential.

- A patient's current appointment and appointment history is confidential.

- Even the information that a person is a patient is confidential.

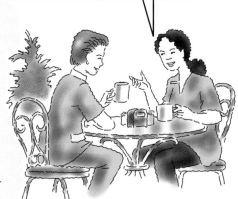

Patient privacy is especially important to remember when spending time with coworkers outside the office. You may want to vent about the difficult patient you dealt with that morning, but remember that's private information.

- storing and managing patients' medical information, such as diagnoses and medical history

Some medical offices began replacing paper medical records with computer records. Health care workers documented patient contacts and treatments with the computer instead of writing in patients' charts.

Government leaders believed that requiring computers to be used in other ways too—such as in dealing with patients' insurance companies—would make health care more efficient. But this proposal increased concerns the public already had about computers. Many people feared that strangers' or criminals' "hacking" their personal information from computers was easier than stealing paper records. Because of such fears, Congress added protections for patients' privacy when it passed HIPAA.

The law itself contains only a few of the privacy requirements you'll read about throughout this book. Instead, Congress empowered the U.S. Department of Health and Human Services (HHS) to issue rules that set the standards for patient privacy. As you learned in Chapter 2, however, administrative rules have the same authority as statutes. They must be obeyed.

THE PRIVACY RULE

The HHS privacy rule is a huge document that greatly affects how a medical office must operate. Here are some of the rule's key provisions that are important for you to know.

- All records containing any items (called "patient identifiers") that could link their contents to a specific patient must be treated as protected health information (PHI).
- Except as required by law or allowed by the privacy rule, PHI may not be disclosed to others without the patient's permission.
- Only the information that is needed should be supplied. For example, if an insurance company is being billed for a specific treatment, only the parts of the medical record related to that treatment should be disclosed.
- Patients have a right to view and receive copies of their own medical records, except in very limited and specific circumstances.
- Patients have a right to know to whom their PHI has been disclosed, except in very limited circumstances.
- Each health care provider must have a privacy notice—a document that states its privacy policies and practices.

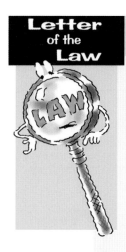

Letter of the Law

HIPAA

The Health Insurance Portability and Accountability Act (HIPAA) of 1996 changed how the health care system operates in four major areas:

1. Transactions
   - creates a single national standard for how diagnoses and treatments are identified and coded on bills for services
   - requires that bills to insurance companies be submitted electronically (by computer)

2. Privacy
   - defines what patient information must be considered private
   - regulates how patient information must be handled and used
   - sets the conditions under which private patient information can be disclosed

3. Security
   - sets standards for protecting patient information that is stored on computers and sent to others electronically, including lab test results and electronic medical records
   - requires the use of passwords, firewalls, antivirus software, and encryption software on computers that contain or transmit patient information

4. Identification
   - creates a national system of codes for identifying individual health care providers, health insurance plans, employers, and patients
   - requires that each provider or health insurance plan include its identifying code on all electronic transmissions

- Each health care provider must train its employees about the HHS privacy rule and appoint a privacy officer to be in charge of its enforcement.

HIPAA and its privacy rule are extremely important and will affect your work as a medical assistant. Because of that, you'll often read about them throughout the rest of this book.

PATIENT IDENTIFIERS

HIPAA recognizes the following items as patient identifiers. If even one of them appears in any patient materials, it makes those materials PHI. Unless all of these identifiers are removed from the information, the privacy rule applies:

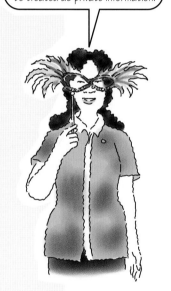

To truly protect a patient's identity, if any of these patient identifiers appears in a patient's medical records, the records must be treated as private information.

- name
- address
- zip code
- phone number
- fax number
- e-mail address
- date of birth
- birth certificate
- Social Security number
- medical record number
- health plan numbers
- driver's license
- vehicle identification number
- license plate number
- website address
- fingerprints and voiceprints
- photos

The Privacy Notice

Patients visiting the office for the first time must receive a copy of the office's privacy notice, stating its policies and practices for protecting patient confidentiality and handling PHI. The notice must contain the following information:

- the ways the office uses PHI—for example, using the patient's phone number to call with appointment reminders—and the patient's right to object to such uses
- the circumstances in which the office may disclose a patient's PHI without obtaining the patient's consent
- the patient's legal rights concerning how his PHI is handled
- the name, address, and phone number of the office's privacy officer, should the patient have any questions or requests

Many offices ask patients to sign a second copy of the privacy notice to show that they received the notice and understand its contents. The signed copy is placed in the patient's record.

When Confidentiality Doesn't Apply

The privacy rule allows providers to release PHI without the patient's permission in the following circumstances:

- to a family member or other individual who is directly responsible for the patient's care, such as in the case of a mentally incompetent adult who is cared for by an adult sister or brother
- to other health care providers who become involved in the patient's care
- to attorneys, public health officials, and law enforcement authorities, where required by court order or state law

These exceptions are generally listed on the privacy notice that providers are required to give to patients. Though it isn't required that a patient sign a consent form for the medical office to obtain payment from a health plan for treatment every time the patient comes in, the patient is required to sign a consent form that allows the medical office to release the patient's information to their insurance company. This consent is signed during the patient's first visit and is valid for that day's visit as well as subsequent visits and treatments.

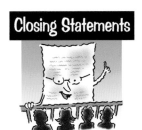

Closing Statements

- A medical assistant's scope of practice is determined by her training and experience, as well as by any state laws that may apply.
- The American Association of Medical Assistants (AAMA) and American Medical Technologists (AMT) maintain lists of knowledge, skills, and duties common to the profession of medical assisting.
- Standard of care is determined by the education and training needed to practice a particular profession. Because physicians have more education and training, they are held to a higher standard of care than medical assistants are.
- Each health care professional is expected to follow orders, be truthful, and generally act as a reasonable member of the profession.
- A harmful act that's purposely committed is called an intentional tort. Many intentional torts are also crimes.

- An unintentional tort is a wrongful act that's committed accidentally, without intent to do harm.
- A person who commits an intentional or unintentional tort is called a tortfeasor.
- Negligence can occur in any of three ways: malfeasance is a wrong and unlawful act; misfeasance is a lawful act performed improperly; and nonfeasance is the failure to perform an act that should have been performed.
- In general, to prove negligence, the injured party must prove that: the tortfeasor owed a *duty* of care; the tortfeasor is guilty of *dereliction of duty* by not providing a proper standard of care; harm or injury was a *direct cause* of that failure of duty; the harm was serious enough to require the tortfeasor to pay *damages* to the injured party.
- HIPAA rules establish which patient information is confidential and when a patient's information may and may not be disclosed. They also require that patients be given a printed notice of the medical office's policies and practices regarding privacy.

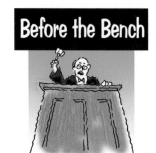

Answer the following multiple-choice questions.

1. The range of activities a medical professional is qualified to perform is called:
   a. scope of practice.
   b. standard of care.
   c. duty of care.
   d. reasonable person standard.

2. According to the AAMA, which of the following is not a common clinical task a medical assistant may be asked to perform?
   a. taking medical histories
   b. removing sutures and changing dressings
   c. performing venipuncture
   d. interpreting test results

3. All of the following determine the standard of care expected from a health care worker *except:*
   a. his medical profession.
   b. the duty of care.
   c. his employer.
   d. the reasonable person standard.

4. To be a tort, an action must:
   a. be intentional.
   b. be unintentional.

    c. result in negligence.

    d. result in harm.

5. What is a tortfeasor?

    a. a victim of a tort

    b. a person who commits a tort

    c. an attorney who sues a physician for a tort

    d. a person who fails to take the proper action

6. In the medical profession, the tort of negligence is known as:

    a. malpractice.

    b. duty of care.

    c. dereliction of duty.

    d. all of the above.

7. A medical professional who does not take an action that's required has failed to meet the requirements of:

    a. scope of practice.

    b. privacy rules.

    c. duty of care.

    d. nonfeasance.

8. If a medical professional commits an intentional tort, she is guilty of:

    a. malpractice.

    b. malfeasance.

    c. a crime.

    d. all of the above

9. Which of the following does *not* have to be proven in a medical malpractice case?

    a. direct or proximate cause

    b. *res ipsa loquitur*

    c. duty of care

    d. the reasonable person standard

10. Which statement about patient confidentiality is *not* true?

    a. Patient consent is always required before a medical office can disclose confidential patient information.

    b. Improper disclosure of confidential patient information is a violation of federal law.

    c. A medical office is required to inform all patients in writing of how it handles confidential patient information.

    d. The fact that a person is a patient of the office is confidential information.

Chapter 4

RISKY BUSINESS: MANAGING RISK AND DEFENSES TO LAWSUITS

Chapter Checklist

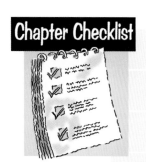

- Explain why quality improvement is important within the medical office

- State why it is necessary to have a risk manager/compliance officer within the office

- Define "burden of knowledge" and describe what to do if you suspect someone in the office has committed malpractice

- List and describe the four Cs of malpractice prevention

- Describe how employees with responsible attitudes can help to decrease the likelihood of the physician being sued

- Explain the importance of continuous staff training

- List the defenses that may be used for professional liability suits

- Explain the importance of professional liability insurance for medical assistants

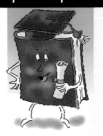

Chapter Competencies

- Perform within legal and ethical boundaries (CAAHEP C.2.b.)

- Project a positive attitude (ABHES 1.a.)

- Be cognizant of ethical boundaries (ABHES 1.d.)

- Evidence a responsible attitude (ABHES 1.g.)

- Perform risk management procedures (ABHES 5.h.)

- Maintain liability coverage (ABHES 6.e.)

In times long past, people sometimes settled disputes with duels. Today, people often settle their disputes with lawsuits. We've all seen the TV ads encouraging viewers with injuries—or possible injuries—to "protect their rights" by calling an attorney, as the lawyer's phone number appears on the screen.

Lawsuits and the fear of being sued have changed the face of health care. Physicians practice medicine differently, and medical offices operate differently as a result. Some changes are probably for the good. Others clearly are not. Malpractice suits are one reason the cost of health care in the United States has increased. They're also a reason that some physicians no longer provide certain services to patients.

You'll learn more about these trends as you read this chapter. You'll also learn how medical offices reduce the risk of being sued, and how these practices affect your job as a medical assistant.

Why People Sue

Compared to the number of patients a medical office sees every week, the number of patients who decide to bring a lawsuit is quite small. However, this small minority of patients can have a long-lasting impact on the daily goings-on in a medical office. Patients sue medical practices and individual health care providers for many reasons. However, the most common reasons can be grouped into two major categories.

- *Medical reasons.* These lawsuits relate directly to the medical treatment the suing patients received. A medical professional may have made a mistake. Or the patient may have suffered an injury or not received the outcome expected.

- *Personal reasons.* These lawsuits relate to a different kind of "treatment"—the manner in which patients are dealt with by the physician and staff. The old saying in health care that "the rude get sued" is generally true! Once again, this is why customer service is vital to the success of the medical practice.

THAT WASN'T SUPPOSED TO HAPPEN!

Of course, treatment errors and other "bad acts" that harm patients can lead to lawsuits. You read about negligence and malpractice in Chapter 3. Other medical factors that can cause patients to sue are:

- poor outcomes
- unrealistic expectations
- poor quality of care

However, in all these cases—and sometimes even with actual malpractice, too—the attitude of the people who work in the practice can make the patient less or more likely to contact an attorney. Sometimes, just acknowledging if you made a small mistake—and saying you're sorry—is all a patient really wants to hear.

Poor Outcomes

The practice of medicine is not an exact science. Patients don't come in with a diagnosis plastered on their foreheads. Unfortunately, the signs and symptoms for one disease can be the signs and symptoms for several diseases. It's up to the physician to determine which disease or ailment the patient is suffering from. Sometimes, despite everyone's best efforts, the result is not what was hoped for or expected. Unless there was malfeasance, misfeasance, or nonfeasance, a bad outcome is not malpractice.

On the other hand, if someone in the office has promised the patient a cure, the patient could argue that a contract had been made. The patient's attorney could then sue—not for malpractice, but for breach of contract. This is one reason why you should never try to reassure a patient by telling him that he's going to be fine.

> Never make any promises to the patient about treatment. This could put you and your office at risk of a lawsuit.

Unrealistic Expectations

Unrealistic expectations are related to poor outcomes. Medical treatments and technology are now so advanced that some patients expect more than is medically possible. Then, when the outcome is not what they expected, they believe they've been treated poorly. This is another reason to avoid telling patients they're going to be okay.

Poor Quality of Care

Sometimes, a health care provider may not meet the duty or standard of care owed to the patient. At other times, the attitudes and behaviors of the provider or of her co-workers may cause the patient to feel that he has not received acceptable care. In either case, a lawsuit may result.

UNDERSTANDING PATIENTS' NEEDS

Patients like to feel that their physician sees them as individuals. That can be a challenge in today's medical world. A physician is more likely to be part of a group practice or a multiphysician clinic. He is also more likely to be a specialist than someone who treats an entire family's illnesses. In addition, some health insurance companies set quotas for the number of patients a physician should see in a day. The close physician-patient relationship of the

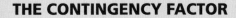

Legal Brief THE CONTINGENCY FACTOR

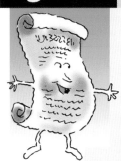

Many patients' attorneys take malpractice suits on **contingency.** This means that the patient does not have to pay the lawyer unless the lawyer wins. The lawyer then gets between 25 and 40 percent of the money the physician must pay.

Some people believe this practice encourages lawsuits because the patient has nothing to lose financially by suing his physician if he's unhappy with his care. Others argue that it discourages such suits because a lawyer will not take a weak case on contingency, since she'll get no money if the patient loses. They also argue that there are people with strong cases who could not afford to sue except on a contingency basis.

On the other hand, the physician's lawyer must be paid whether the physician wins or loses. This causes physicians to sometimes settle even weak malpractice suits out of court if the settlement amount is less than the cost of a trial. In such cases, the patient's lawyer gets her contingency fee from the settlement paid to the patient.

past is now largely gone. Today, some patients fear that their physician views them not as people, but as conditions, diseases, or one more patient toward the daily or monthly quota.

But What About Me?

A physician's office can be a busy place with a hectic schedule. Medical assistants want to move quickly to get patients into the treatment rooms and then on to x-ray or the lab for tests, or out the door. Sometimes, physicians may see four to six patients an hour, which leaves little time for small talk.

This frantic pace can make patients feel frustrated—and even angry—about being treated with so little apparent regard. The patient may interpret the physician's casual attitude as a lack of caring or empathy. If the physician's hurried schedule leaves the patient with unanswered questions or unexpressed concerns, the patient's frustration may be even greater.

It's your job as a medical assistant to help make up for what the patient may view as the physician's failing in this area. Showing empathy and caring will be an important part of your job—whether that patient feels rushed by the physician or upset by office delays.

The secret is in communication. You'll read more on this subject later in this chapter. For now, just remember that patients who are upset over how they are treated are more likely to sue if they're unsatisfied with their medical care.

Common Complaints

Surveys of patients consistently show that problems with even getting to see a physician are a major source of frustration. These delays and scheduling problems cause headaches for both staff and patients.

The Scheduling Crisis

Patients complain about long waits in scheduling appointments. People who aren't feeling well understandably want to get treatment so they will feel better. They are often frustrated that their illness might worsen before their appointment date arrives.

While scheduling appointments will always be a challenge, it's a good idea to leave some open slots for emergencies. Also, always keep a positive attitude when trying to manage difficult schedules with patients.

I understand that you're not feeling well. Let's see what we can do to get you in tomorrow morning.

The Physician Will Be with You Shortly . . .

Often, patients must sit in waiting rooms for a long time. The physician may be behind schedule, and there may be good reasons for the delay. However, long waits make patients feel unimportant and that the office has little concern for their own schedule and inconvenience. Keep patients updated about the status of their appointments, and be realistic about the time. As a medical assistant, do what you can to make their waiting time as pleasant as possible.

Offer the patients options when the physician is running behind. If possible, contact the patient before he leaves work or home and let him know that the physician is running an hour behind. This allows the patient to come in an hour later or reschedule his appointment. If you're unable to contact the patient prior to the appointment, let him know when he arrives. You may suggest that he wait in the office in case the physician catches up, or you may suggest that the patient return at a certain time or reschedule the appointment if desired. When you offer patients options, they are less likely to become agitated because they're taking part in the decisionmaking process.

The Trouble with Overbooking

Some offices "double-book" two patients into the same time slot or schedule all the patients the physician will see during an hour at the same time. This can cause long delays for some patients. It can also lead to a very crowded waiting room. If this happens frequently in your medical office, the staff might want to brainstorm more effective ways to schedule patient appointments.

Managing Risk

You won't be alone in your efforts to prevent lawsuits. Most medical offices follow practices that are designed to reduce the risk of injury to patients and employees—and therefore the risk of lawsuits. This activity is known as **risk management.**

THE RISK MANAGER'S DUTIES

A risk manager or compliance officer usually organizes the office's risk management program. Her job is to coordinate the various parts of the program and make sure that each part or portion is being carried out.

The risk management process involves identifying possible dangers and other problems and then taking steps to prevent or eliminate them. There are several basic parts of an effective risk management program.

Name That Job Description

Every position in a medical office should have a written job description. It should list:

- the position's responsibilities
- the tasks to be performed by the employee who holds the position

Some job descriptions also list the skills required for the position. See the sample job description below.

MEDICAL ASSISTANT JOB DESCRIPTION

What is the chief objective of this position?

The chief objective of this position is to provide clinical and administrative support to the medical office and the patients the office serves. In this capacity, the incumbent is constantly exposed to internal and external scrutiny, stresses, ambiguities, and confidential patient information. Therefore, the employee must respond to these conditions in a professionally acceptable manner.

What knowledge, skills, and abilities should an employee bring to this position?

Current clinical and administrative support experience:

- knowledge of the principles and skills needed for clinical care to provide care and treatment
- knowledge of examination, diagnostic, and treatment room procedures
- knowledge of medications and their effects on patients
- knowledge of common safety hazards and precautions to establish a safe work environment
- skill in using various types of equipment for examination and treatment procedures
- skill in taking vital signs
- skill in maintaining records

Administrative skills:

- skill in answering the phone in the proper manner and scheduling patients for various appointments within the office as well as outside appointments, including hospital admissions

- knowledge of basic bookkeeping
- knowledge of basic insurance terms and procedures needed to provide patients with the correct information regarding their coverage
- knowledge of HIPAA
- basic computer skills

Interpersonal skills:

- skill in establishing and maintaining effective working relationships with patients, medical staff, and the public
- ability to maintain quality control standards
- ability to recognize problems and recommend solutions
- ability to react calmly and effectively in emergency situations
- ability to interpret, adapt, and apply guidelines and procedures
- ability to communicate clearly with excellent verbal and written communications skills and experience in clinical documentation
- ability to organize tasks and manage time effectively
- ability to work with a minimum of supervision
- ability to respond efficiently and calmly in a medical emergency
- ability to interact effectively with people of diverse backgrounds and temperaments
- patience during times of stress

Level and type of experience:

- a minimum of graduation from an accredited Medical Assisting curriculum (two years of experience in a physician practice setting preferred)

Education or training (cite major area of study):

- Graduation from an accredited Medical Assisting program required
- Must have valid certification or registration as a medical assistant and current provider CPR certification

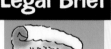 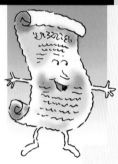

Legal Brief   THE LAW OF AGENCY

The **law of agency** controls the relationship that is formed when one person agrees to perform work for another person. It makes an employee the "agent" of her employer and the employer therefore legally responsible for her actions. This is the principle on which the doctrine of *respondeat superior* is based.

The law of agency works best when there's a written job description that clearly defines the employee's duties. As long as the employee performs only those duties, she is protected by the law of agency. But, if her actions are not part of her job description, then the law of agency and *respondeat superior* do not apply.

How Should I Do This Again?

The risk manager or compliance office is responsible for maintaining a **procedures manual**. A separate, written, step-by-step procedure should exist for every clinical and administrative task performed in the office. Following set procedures reduces the risk of misfeasance. Copies of the manual should be available for employees to refer to, if necessary.

Know the Policies

A **policy manual** consists of general statements of the office's practices, standards, and goals in basic areas of operation, including:

- patient privacy
- clinical treatment
- patient communications
- documentation

The tasks described in the procedures manual should be aimed at carrying out the policies in the policy manual.

QUALITY IMPROVEMENT

Quality improvement (QI)—also called quality assurance (QA)—is the measures an office takes to help guarantee a high quality of patient care. In many offices, the risk manager or compliance officer is responsible for the QI program. In many practices, the office manager takes on these responsibilities. His responsibilities can be broad and include the following:

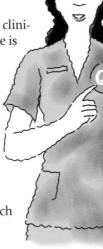

Quality is important!

- making sure that all government regulations are being followed
- monitoring office activities to be sure that proper procedures are being followed
- monitoring the checking of all administrative, clinical, and lab equipment to make sure they are working properly
- making sure that the drugs, other medications, and clinical supplies being used are not out of date and there is proper disposal if any are found to be out of date
- ensuring that all biohazard waste is disposed of properly
- arranging for or monitoring the continuing education and training of staff to make sure they're current on the skills and knowledge they need to do their jobs including annual training on bloodborne pathogens and current CPR certification for necessary staff
- maintaining the office itself so that no hazards, such as broken furniture or frayed electrical cords, can injure patients or employees

DEFENSIVE MEDICINE

Risk management shapes the way physicians practice medicine. Some physicians now order more lab tests, x-rays, consultations, and referrals than they did in the past. They want to make sure their diagnoses are accurate and that no one can sue them for missing something they should have caught. As you read earlier, all this fear and extra precautions contribute to the rising cost of health care.

Another result of defensive medicine is increased specialization. Fewer general practitioners are willing to deliver babies or fix broken bones. Even many Ob/Gyn physicians have given up the *obstetrics* (childbirth) part of their practice because the risks of being sued are greater than for the gynecology part of their practice. (*Gynecology* is the treatment of the female reproductive system.)

Avoiding Risk

Physicians sometimes refuse to accept new patients with serious or complicated problems. Some refer treatment of these patients to other, more highly specialized physicians. Physicians may also be unwilling to try new treatments, procedures, or drugs. Why?

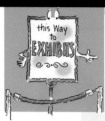

WHEN BAD THINGS HAPPEN

If a patient is injured or you make a treatment mistake, it's important to follow proper procedures.

1. Your first action should be to tell the physician immediately, if she is available, or your supervisor, so that any possibly harmful effects of the event can be dealt with.

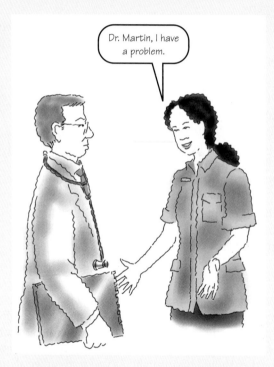

2. Most offices also require that such events be reported on forms called **incident reports.** You'll be asked to write a description of what happened, what was said and by whom, and who else witnessed the event. It's important that you only document your own conversations and actions; you should never write an incident report documenting someone else's experience!

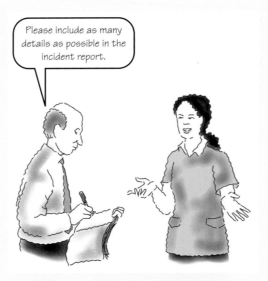

3. You should avoid making statements about what
   caused the event or what (or whom) is to blame.
   Your task is to state the facts only, without providing
   your opinions, theories, or conclusion.

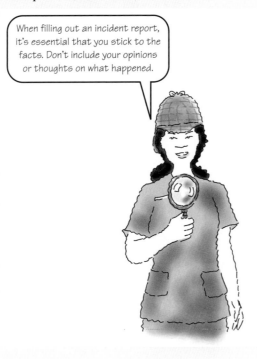

4. Be cautious in discussing the event with the patient. Never state or hint at who or what you think might be responsible, or that a mistake was made. Also, avoid any response that might suggest you agree or disagree with the patient's version of the event.

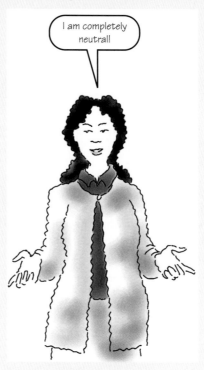

They fear the possible legal consequences if the outcome is poor. A wall of suspicion and mistrust has grown between many physicians and patients.

The Conspiracy of Silence

It's difficult or impossible in many situations to find a physician who's willing to testify in court against another physician in a malpractice suit. Some physicians have pity on their colleagues and picture themselves in the place of the accused. Others fear that they'll be outcasts in the medical profession if they testify against other physicians. So, they remain silent.

By the Book — CALL IN THE CHAPERONES

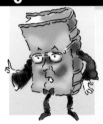

One way that medical offices sometimes manage risk is by using chaperones when a physician examines a patient, generally those of the opposite sex. It may be one of your duties as a medical assistant to be a chaperone in certain circumstances. This means that you'll remain in the room while the physician conducts the examination.

Chaperones aren't just for school dances! The physician may call on you to be a chaperone, or witness, during an examination as added protection.

Chaperones usually are the same gender as the patient. But, if necessary, a chaperone of the opposite gender (that is, the same gender as the physician) may be used. The idea is to have a third person present to guard against any claims by the patient that the physician behaved improperly. If the patient has brought someone to accompany them into the room, that person does not count as the third person. If a lawsuit were to arise, the patient's friend or family member would likely side with the patient, leaving the medical office no protection.

AN OUNCE OF PREVENTION . . .

Like any business, a medical practice must ensure that its premises are safe. (**Premises** are the building and grounds, or the part of a building, where the business is conducted.) No hazards should exist that might injure customers or employees.

Managing premises risk is especially important for a medical office. That's because many of your patients may have medical conditions that increase their chances for accident and injury. All employees are responsible for reporting or correcting hazards that could cause injuries.

Ethics in Action   THE BURDEN OF KNOWLEDGE

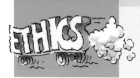

Despite the conspiracy of silence, you have a responsibility to come forward if you're aware of wrong-doing in the office. It's a violation of professional ethics and your duty of care if you don't do so. In ethics, your duty to speak out in such situations is known as the burden (duty) of knowledge. That means if you know something went wrong, you have an ethical duty to reveal it.

> The duty to do something unpleasant can be a real burden sometimes!

As a medical assistant, you may be greeting patients as they arrive or escorting them to treatment rooms. Here are some things you can do.

- Pay special attention to your work area.
- Be on the lookout for waiting room hazards, such as broken chairs or magazines that have fallen on the floor, where patients might slip on them or injure themselves.
- If you're working as a receptionist, walking though the waiting room several times a day to look for hazards is a good risk management behavior.

MANAGING PRODUCT RISKS

Medical offices use drugs, medicines, and other products that can have side effects. Some also may have a potential for harm if used improperly. In either case, providers owe a duty of care to use the products correctly and to warn patients of possible side effects. They also have a duty to instruct on proper use of products they send patients home with. "Failure to warn" is a major cause of lawsuits!

For example, suppose you administer a medication to a patient that can make her drowsy. But you fail to warn her of this possible side effect and don't caution her about driving. If she falls asleep while driving home and gets into an accident, she can sue you and your employer.

In one case, a medical office sent a patient home with some chemical heat packs to use on his sore muscles. But office employees failed to tell him how to use the pack properly. So he applied it directly to his skin, without placing a towel as insulation. The patient suffered serious burns as a result. The court found the medical office **liable,** or legally responsible, for the injury.

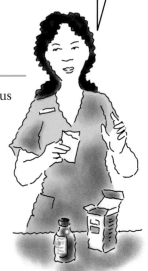

Read package inserts! It's your duty to know the proper uses, risks, and side effects of products you use or supply to patients.

Practicing Preventive Medicine

Preventive medicine includes medical practices that focus on *preventing* diseases instead of just curing them. But there's another way to think of preventive medicine, too. That's practicing medicine in a way that will prevent lawsuits.

The key to this kind of preventive medicine is behavior. That means treating patients in ways that reduce their anxiety and frustration with the situation. It means showing the right attitude—cheerful, helpful, understanding, and professional. And showing a professional attitude includes how you treat your job as well as how you treat patients.

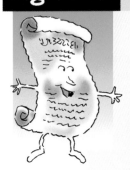

Legal Brief   EQUIPMENT FAILURES

Some malpractice suits have been based on charges that office equipment didn't work properly. Equipment failures include machines that break, causing injury to the patient. Another risk is improperly functioning machines that produce inaccurate results. For example, a glucose meter reports a falsely low glucose level in a patient's blood, causing the physician to miss a diagnosis of diabetes.

Courts have ruled that a medical office is responsible for having equipment that is safe and working properly. This is why OSHA requires documentation in various logs to show you have run controls on such equipment. However, the reasonable person standard also applies. If the defect was not apparent to reasonable inspection, the office is not liable for any harm the equipment caused. The equipment's manufacturer or servicer may be liable, however.

Every employee of a medical office has a responsibility to act in ways that help prevent lawsuits or that make any suits that *are* filed less likely to succeed. In fact, risk management includes four areas of behavior that are known as the four Cs of malpractice prevention.

- *Caring.* A sincere concern for patients is probably the most important attitude you can show.
- *Communication.* Being a good communicator will help you gain patients' trust and respect.
- *Charting.* A patient's medical record is important evidence that can help defend against lawsuits.
- *Competence.* Knowing and following the requirements of good medical practice will help you provide patients with a high standard of care.

I CARE!

Communication is the key to showing patients that you care. It includes how you listen as well as what you say and how you say it. Your attitude, behaviors, and body language are also forms of communication.

Genuine caring requires that you communicate three things to patients:

- understanding
- empathy
- compassion

Understanding

Caring involves showing patients that you understand. It means that you're aware patients may be anxious, fearful, angry, frustrated, or filled with a variety of other emotions that often accompany having a medical problem. Understanding also involves showing patients that you recognize and value their points of view.

Empathy

Showing that you care also includes showing empathy. You read about empathy in Chapter 1. It's a form of communication that's deeper than understanding. Empathy involves sharing the patient's feeling rather than just understanding him. It's the ability to imagine what it would be like to actually *be* that patient, with all that he's going through.

Compassion

Compassion is a desire to help others. It's one more step beyond understanding and empathy. A compassionate health care provider not only understands and feels the patient's "pain," he tries to ease that "pain." It's the final step in caring. But remember, while it's important to help a patient feel better, it's also important to avoid making any promises about her medical condition or treatment.

I feel your pain. I'll do what I can to help.

CASUAL, CARING, AND CONCERNED

You don't want to be uptight or appear overly serious. Communicating these attitudes can make you seem cold and unapproachable or make the patient more anxious. You want to be friendly and casual with patients, but not too casual. Many patients view an overly casual attitude as a lack of concern. In either case, when patients view health care workers as cold, unconcerned, or uncaring, they are more likely to sue if something goes wrong.

Caring and Co-workers

Remember that your attitudes and behaviors with co-workers are as important as those you have with patients. Avoid inappropriate or unprofessional behavior anywhere in the office. This includes:

- loud laughing
- horseplay
- displays of secrecy or extreme excitement

Also, never criticize another health care worker in front of patients. Likewise, never criticize another medical practice or physician in front of a patient. Remember, if patients see you acting one way with co-workers and another way with them, they may question whether your caring attitude is genuine and sincere.

LET'S TALK

Patients who view a medical office's workers as friendly and helpful are less likely to sue. You can help create this feeling by using good listening skills and other good communication techniques.

By the Book   COMMUNICATION GUIDELINES

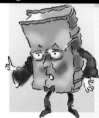

Here are some communication guidelines that will help prevent lawsuits.

- Maintain the privacy of all conversations with patients. Never discuss patient information in front of other patients.
- Put all special instructions for patients in writing.
- Return patients' phone calls as soon as possible. Give patients emergency phone numbers to use when the office is closed.
- Listen carefully to all patients' remarks, concerns, and complaints and take them seriously. Report them to the appropriate office employees.
- Learn to recognize when the symptoms patients report require the physician's immediate attention and when patients should be told to seek emergency care.
- Discuss fees and payment policies with the patient before treatment begins.

For example, sitting rather than standing when you talk with a patient communicates the attitude that you care and are interested in what the patient has to say.

It's important that patients never feel hurried or "brushed off" when they talk with you. They need to feel that the time you give them is not rushed. Making eye contact as you talk also communicates your attention and interest. The use of appropriate touch, such as a hand on the shoulder or forearm, also indicates genuine concern.

IF IT'S NOT IN THE CHART . . .

Another way to practice "preventive medicine" and avoid lawsuits is to be sure that patients' charts are accurate. Patient records are often used as evidence in malpractice suits. Improper or insufficient documentation could cause the office to lose a malpractice case.

Each patient's medical record should clearly show:

- what procedures and other treatments the patient received and when each was done, including the date and time of each procedure

- all test results
- medications prescribed, including refills

This information is needed to show that nothing was overlooked or neglected in caring for the patient, and that the patient's care clearly met the standards required by law.

You'll read more about documentation and patient records in Chapter 7. But here are some areas that need special attention to manage risks and defend against possible lawsuits.

Patient Contacts

All patient contacts should be documented in the chart. This includes documenting all calls made to or received from the patient, with a summary of their content. If the patient is discussing symptoms or complaints, try to document her exact words if possible. Use quotation marks when documenting to show exactly what the patient has told you.

Missed Appointments

You should attempt to contact all patients who miss an appointment or cancel it without rescheduling. Document these calls and their outcome in the patients' charts. Also indicate "no show," "cancelled," or "cancelled and rescheduled" in the office appointment log and keep these records.

Referrals

If the physician refers the patient to another physician, clarify whether your office will schedule the appointment or if the patient is to schedule the appointment. Make sure the patient understands how to proceed and document it in the chart. If the office makes the appointment, record the appointment time and date in the chart and note that the patient agreed to it. If the patient is to schedule the appointment, provide her with all information about that practice, including the phone number, contact person, and address.

In either case, follow up with a phone call to the other physician's office to make sure the appointment was kept. Document the call in the chart. Note whether a report was received from the other physician, and document her recommendations for further care of the patient.

Consent and Refusal

Make sure that each patient's record contains the signed and dated consent forms necessary for treatment. If a patient refuses an examination, treatment, or test, document the patient's refusal in his chart. If possible, have the patient sign a statement that he's refusing and place the statement in his chart.

It's your ethical duty as a professional to have the knowledge and skills you need to do your job. Remaining competent means updating old knowledge, procedures, behaviors, and skills to keep up with changes in the office or in the general practice of medicine. Your employer will expect this of you and, in many cases, may require it.

Professional Competence

There are several ways you can keep up with current developments and show competence in your profession, such as:

- reading journals and newsletters
- interacting with other medical assistants
- obtaining or maintaining credentials as a Certified Medical Assistant (CMA) through the AAMA or a Registered Medical Assistant (RMA) through the AMT

Many employers offer staff training. You should make the most of these opportunities, even if doing so is not required. Voluntary attendance is further evidence of your professionalism and desire to improve your knowledge and skills.

Colleges, professional associations, and other organizations offer many educational opportunities outside the office. Attending professional meetings, conferences, and noncredit classes are excellent ways of keeping your skills and knowledge up to date. Employers will often pay the costs of this continuing education.

Workplace Competence

Being a competent professional requires a good knowledge of your field. This knowledge adds to your competence in the workplace by making you more aware of your abilities and limitations.

Know the requirements of good medical care for each patient, but always work within your scope of practice. Never try to do something that you're not trained to do.

BEHAVIORS THAT REDUCE RISK

Here are some everyday behaviors that will reduce your employer's risk of being sued.

- Always act within your scope of practice.
- Keep equipment in safe and working order and ready to use.

- Keep floors clean and clear.
- Open doors carefully.
- Dispose of biohazardous waste in the proper containers.
- Thoroughly document all contact with patients.
- Never promise a recovery or cure.
- Maintain the confidentiality of all patient information.
- Acknowledge long waits and give patients a reason for their wait.
- Treat all patients with courtesy and respect.

By the Book — MAKING SURE YOU KNOW

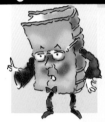

In a busy medical practice it's easy to imagine how a hurried provider might give a wrong treatment to a wrong patient. However, there are standard procedures to prevent this from happening.

- When you prepare a medication for a patient, check it three times. Check it first when you take it from the supply cabinet, again when you prepare the dose, and a third time when you return the container to the shelf.

- Always look for the patient's name and date of birth on his chart or on the physician's order for a treatment or medication. Instead of asking, "Are you John Smith?" ask the patient to state his name and date of birth. It's possible that the patient is not listening and will answer in the affirmative. But if you have him tell you his name and possibly another identifying mark such as date of birth or Social Security number, you can be sure you have the correct person. Make sure the physician's order and the patient match before giving the treatment or medication. If they don't, stop and make sure you've got the right patient!

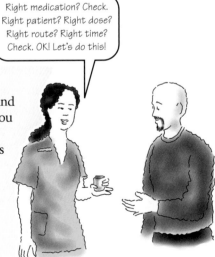

Right medication? Check. Right patient? Right dose? Right route? Right time? Check. OK! Let's do this!

A Good Defense Is the Best Offense

You've been reading in this chapter about ways to manage risks and avoid lawsuits. But lawsuits happen! And when patients sue, health care providers can defend themselves in a number of ways.

There are three main kinds of defenses:

- assertions of innocence
- technical defenses
- affirmative defenses

The innocence defense denies that wrongdoing took place. If any of the patient's charges are true, this defense won't work. Another defense will have to be used.

TECHNICAL DEFENSES

Technical defenses are defenses that depend on legal points and principles rather than on the evidence and facts in the case. Here are four technical defenses that might be used against a malpractice suit:

- the statute of limitations
- release of tortfeasor
- *res judicata*
- the borrowed servant doctrine

The Statute of Limitations

Probably the first thing the defense attorney will investigate is whether the statute of limitations has expired on the alleged wrongdoing. As you read in Chapter 2, the statute of limitations is a state law that limits the length of time a plaintiff has to bring charges. That time limit generally depends on three things:

- the state in which the alleged wrongdoing took place
- whether the alleged wrongdoing violated civil law or criminal law
- the specific type of wrongdoing involved

In most states, the time limit for filing malpractice suits is two years. But as you read in Chapter 2, that time limit can vary in some states if the patient is a child or if the injury takes time to appear.

Release of Tortfeasor

As you learned in Chapter 3, a tortfeasor is someone who is guilty of committing a tort. Release of tortfeasor is a legal doctrine that often applies in situations where there's more than one tortfeasor.

Legal Brief — THE STATUTE OF LIMITATIONS AND MEDICAL ASSISTANTS

Time limits for filing malpractice suits are often longer than those for filing ordinary negligence suits. Both can apply to the actions of a medical assistant. If the medical assistant's alleged wrongdoing involves clinical duties, the longer time limits on malpractice may apply. On the other hand, receptionist and administrative duties are not viewed as professional activities. So, wrongdoing in these areas is not considered malpractice. Therefore, the shorter time limits attached to negligence would apply.

Suppose a driver injures someone in an auto accident. The physician makes a medical mistake when treating the victim. In most states, the driver is liable for any harm caused by the physician's malpractice. That's because the driver was responsible for the victim's need to go to the physician in the first place.

If the victim sues the driver for the injuries, the victim can't collect damages from the physician, too. That's because the money the driver must pay the victim also releases the physician from liability. The physician would use this release of tortfeasor defense if the victim tries to sue her.

Res Judicata

Res judicata is a legal doctrine that a claim can't be retried once a lawsuit has been decided or settled. It's a Latin term that means "the thing has been decided." For example, if a physician is found innocent of a wrongdoing in a lawsuit, the patient can't bring the same suit with a different attorney based on the same evidence.

Here's another example of *res judicata*. Suppose a patient didn't pay his bill. When the physician sues him, his defense for not paying is that the physician was negligent. If the physician wins her suit, the patient can't turn around and sue the physician for negligence. That's because the negligence issue has already been decided in the physician's favor. It was determined when the jury in the physician's suit rejected the patient's defense for not paying his bill.

Borrowed Servant Doctrine

The **borrowed servant doctrine** is the legal principle that releases an employer from liability for an employee's actions if the employee is working for someone else. For example, suppose your employer asks you to help out at a nearby practice that's currently understaffed. If you make a treatment error at the other practice, your employer can't be held responsible for your wrongdoing.

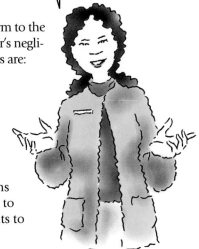

The borrowed servant doctrine is an exception to the doctrine of respondeat superior.

AFFIRMATIVE DEFENSES

Affirmative defenses present evidence that the harm to the patient was due to a reason other than the provider's negligence. The four most common affirmative defenses are:

- contributory negligence
- comparative negligence
- assumption of risk
- emergency

Contributory Negligence

Contributory negligence is a defense that claims the patient's own actions caused or contributed to his injury. Even if the health care provider admits to

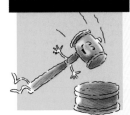

What's the Verdict?   WHO'S RESPONSIBLE?

A medical assistant gave a patient a medication and failed to warn him of its possible side effects. Soon after returning home, he developed a reaction to the drug. A rash appeared all over his body, and he began to have difficulty breathing. Over the next few hours, his breathing difficulties increased. Finally, he went into respiratory arrest and died. The patient's family sued the medical office for negligence and wrongful death because of the medical assistant's failure to warn the patient.

The Verdict: The medical assistant should have alerted the patient to the drug's possible side effects. But the patient was also negligent because he never called the office after experiencing problems. A reasonable person would have recognized a possible connection between receiving a medication and severe symptoms that develop soon after receiving it and would have called the office to report a problem. Had the patient done that, medical intervention could have prevented his death. The medical assistant was negligent in failing to warn the patient. However, a contributory negligence defense would be effective against the wrongful death claim.

negligence, if she can prove that the patient was also partly at fault, the patient can't collect damages.

Comparative Negligence

Comparative negligence also argues that the patient was partly responsible for his injury. But unlike contributory negligence, this defense allows the patient to recover damages based on how much of the injury was not his fault.

For example, suppose a medical assistant accidentally cut a patient's arm. She bandaged the arm and told the patient to replace the bandage with a new one every day. The patient failed to do that, and the cut became infected. If the patient is suing for $100,000 and the court determines he was 60 percent responsible for his injury, $40,000 is the most he can collect if the medical assistant is found negligent.

> This defense may not work if the bad outcome was caused by a treatment error.

Assumption of Risk

Assumption of Risk

Assumption of risk is a defense based on the claim that the patient knew the risks involved in the treatment when she agreed to go ahead with it. To succeed with this defense, the provider must prove *both* of the following circumstances.

- The patient was aware of the risk of bad outcomes.
- Those bad outcomes were the cause of the patient's injury.

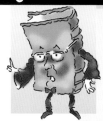

By the Book   OBTAINING INFORMED CONSENT

Proving assumption of risk is much easier if the patient has signed a consent form that lists the risks involved in the treatment. The patient must be aware of the risks of having the procedure, the risks of *not* having the procedure, and any alternative procedures that may exist. A patient's agreement to a treatment after being educated about its possible benefits and risks is called **informed consent.**

Obtaining informed consent is the physician's responsibility. It's not your job as a medical assistant. However, a medical assistant does owe a duty of care to the physician to make sure that properly signed and dated consent forms are in the patient's chart before the treatment is performed. Often, the physician will ask the medical assistant to witness a signature.

Emergency

Emergency is an affirmative defense in which the provider claims that the care was given during an emergency situation and should therefore not be held to as high a standard as non-emergency care. To succeed, this defense must prove the following.

- A true emergency existed.
- The emergency situation was not caused by the provider's actions.
- The standard of care was appropriate for an emergency situation.

Malpractice Insurance: A Good Investment

Another way that medical providers manage risks is by carrying liability and malpractice insurance. Then, if they are successfully sued, the insurance company pays the damages to the patient. In most cases, the insurance company will also pay the costs of defending the provider against the suit.

A medical office's liability and malpractice insurance usually covers its employees' actions in carrying out their duties. However, many medical assistants also obtain their own insurance. Why do they do this?

Sometimes, in a lawsuit, the parties being sued may not all agree on the best course of action. If the patient has sued both the medical assistant and the medical assistant's employer for malpractice, the defense the employer pursues may not be best for the medical assistant.

For example, the employer may decide that it's less expensive to settle a case out of court by admitting to employee wrongdoing when in fact the employee did nothing wrong. If this happens, the medical assistant may want to have his own attorney and defend himself separately from his employer.

Malpractice insurance can be expensive. But it's likely to cost less than having to hire your own attorney and pay damages yourself if you lose your case. For this reason, many medical assistants view having their own malpractice insurance as a wise investment.

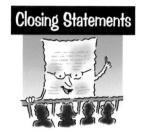

Closing Statements

- Medical reasons for lawsuits include poor treatment outcomes, unrealistic expectations for outcomes, and the belief that suing patients have received poor care.
- Patients are more likely to sue when they feel ignored or mistreated. Long delays in seeing the physician add to their feelings of frustration.
- Written job descriptions, procedures and policy manuals, and quality assurance programs are all devices that offices use to help limit problems that can cause lawsuits. Offices also manage risk by practicing defensive medicine, eliminating premises hazards, and reducing harm from misuse of medications and faulty equipment.
- You can help your employer prevent lawsuits by following the four Cs of malpractice prevention: *caring* for patients; having good *communication* skills; making sure *charting* is thorough and accurate; and achieving *competence* by continuing to update skills and by following proper procedures.
- Technical defenses against lawsuits depend on legal points and principles rather than on the facts and evidence in the case. They include the statute of limitations, the release of tortfeasor defense, the doctrine of *res judicata,* and the borrowed servant doctrine.
- Affirmative defenses against lawsuits are based on presenting evidence that some factor other than negligence caused the patient's injury. Common affirmative defenses include contributory negligence, comparative negligence, assumption of risk, and that an emergency situation existed.
- Most employers' malpractice policies cover their employees. However, the possibly conflicting goals of the employer and the medical assistant in such suits make malpractice insurance for medical assistants a good idea.

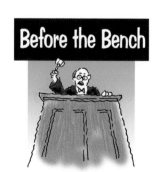

Before the Bench

Answer the following multiple-choice questions.

1. Which factor can cause a patient to sue a medical office?
   a. a poor outcome in the treatment of the patient
   b. the patient's unreasonable expectations for a cure
   c. the patient's frustration with experiences with the office
   d. all of the above

2. Which of the following is *not* part of a good risk management plan?
   a. a written job description for every employee
   b. a conspiracy of silence
   c. a procedures manual
   d. a quality improvement program

3. Who is usually responsible for making sure a medical office's quality improvement plan is effective?
   a. the risk manager
   b. the physician
   c. the medical assistant
   d. all of the above

4. A health care worker's ethical responsibility to speak up when she is aware of wrongdoing is known as:
   a. the burden of knowledge.
   b. assumption of risk.
   c. the borrowed servant doctrine.
   d. contributory negligence.

5. Which is *not* one of the four Cs of malpractice prevention?
   a. charting
   b. communication
   c. confidentiality
   d. caring

6. Which characteristic suggests that a health care worker is a competent professional?
   a. She always carries out the instructions of her supervisor.
   b. She keeps current on new developments in her field.
   c. She is willing to work outside her scope of practice.
   d. all of the above

7. The key employee behavior for reducing the risk that patients will file lawsuits is:
   a. good communication.
   b. showing empathy.
   c. thorough documentation.
   d. respecting confidentiality.

8. Which of the following is *not* an affirmative defense against lawsuits?
   a. emergency
   b. comparative negligence
   c. contributory negligence
   d. assertion of innocence

9. Which of the following is *not* a technical defense against lawsuits?
   a. the statute of limitations
   b. the borrowed servant doctrine
   c. assumption of risk
   d. *res judicata*

10. Why might a medical assistant want to purchase his own professional liability insurance?
    a. because the liability insurance of most medical offices doesn't cover medical assistants
    b. because in defending against a lawsuit, his best interests and those of his employer may not be the same
    c. because his employer's liability insurance may not pay for his legal defense
    d. because the damages awarded to the patient may exceed the limits on the employer's liability insurance policy

Chapter 5

THE LETTER
OF THE LAW:
MEDICAL LAWS
AND STATUTES

Chapter Checklist

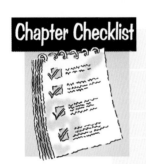

- Discuss the difference between licensure, certification, and registration and how each is maintained

- Explain why it is illegal for medical assistants to call themselves nurses

- Discuss the process of medical legislation

- Describe the process of becoming a physician, including board certification

- Explain the difference between reciprocity and endorsement

- List four reasons physicians may lose their license

- Describe the process a physician goes through to obtain and maintain a DEA license

- Differentiate between fraud and abuse

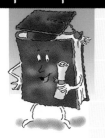

Chapter Competencies

- Perform within legal and ethical boundaries (CAAHEP 3.c.2.b.)

- Demonstrate knowledge of federal and state health-care legislation and regulations (CAAHEP 3.c.2.e.)

- Conduct work within scope of education, training, and ability (ABHES 1.i.)

- Professional components (ABHES 2.p.)

- Allied health professions and credentialing (ABHES 2.q.)

- Maintain licenses and accreditation (ABHES 5.f.)

To assure a high standard of health care, states have long licensed their major practitioners—physicians and nurses. Over time, however, the practice of medicine has come to depend on a team of other health care professionals. To help maintain quality of care, states and professional groups have established standards for these workers, too. In this chapter, you'll learn about these standards, some important laws that control how medicine is practiced, and other laws that are likely to directly affect your activities as a medical assistant.

Modern Medicine

As you read in Chapter 4, the day of the family doctor—the sole practitioner who saw all kinds of patients with the help of a receptionist and maybe an office nurse—is largely gone. In most places, the single physician has been replaced by group practices and large, multispecialty clinics. Often, hospitals own these group practices, which allows the practice to offer employees hospital benefits such as education reimbursement and, many times, better insurance. Group practices can be as small as three physicians, or they may involve a large number of physicians.

Unlike physicians in clinics, the physicians in a group practice generally all have the same specialty. That is, they all practice the same type of medicine. Some examples of medical specialties are *cardiology* (the treatment of diseases of the heart and blood vessels), *oncology* (the treatment of cancerous and noncancerous tumors), and *pediatrics* (the treatment of children).

Not only have physicians become more specialized, the other workers who assist in the practice of medicine have become more specialized, too. They can be classified into two general types:

- **allied health professionals**—people who are licensed, certified, or registered to practice their job or profession
- **paraprofessionals**—people who are trained to assist in the practice of medicine without any license, certification, or registration

LICENSING

A **license** is legal permission required to practice an occupation. State laws usually determine the requirements necessary to practice the occupation. For example, in most cases, a physician must be licensed by the state in order to practice medicine in that state. To practice the profession without a license is against the law. Severe penalties, including large fines and jail time, will result.

Who Needs a License?

It's not just physicians that need a license to practice. In most states, other examples of professionals that require licenses include the following:

- dentists
- pharmacists
- architects
- accountants
- engineers

In general, the occupations that require licenses are those that could cause great harm if untrained and incompetent people are carrying out these tasks. Licensing is designed to protect the public by setting standards that must be met before a person may qualify to perform those occupations. For example, think of the harm that could result if a skyscraper or a bridge is designed by an unqualified architect or engineer. Think about the mess an unqualified accountant could make of a business's finances and operations.

Licensing in the Medical Office

You'll read shortly about how physicians are licensed to practice medicine. But here are some other licensed persons you're likely to find in a large medical office or clinic.

Registered Nurse

Despite the title "registered," a *registered nurse* (RN) is a licensed professional. Some states also license advanced practice nurses. They are highly skilled nurses who have a master's degree in nursing (MSN).

Licensed Practical Nurse

A *licensed practical nurse (LPN)* is licensed to perform some, but not all, of the tasks of a registered nurse. In some states, a licensed practical nurse is also called a licensed vocational nurse (LVN).

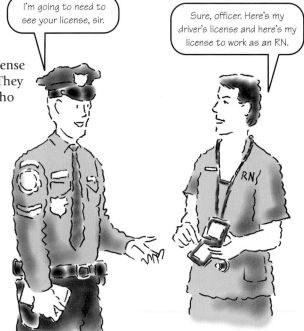

Physician Assistant

A *physician assistant (PA)* performs some physician duties under a physician's supervision. Physician assistants can legally perform more tasks than registered nurses. Some states license physician assistants, while others require certification or registration. Depending upon the state, some physician assistants can also write prescriptions and assist in surgery.

Nurse Practitioner

Registered nurses with advanced education and training in diagnosis and certain other areas of medicine can be licensed as *nurse practitioners* (NPs). Nurse practitioners can perform certain tasks without being under the supervision of a physician. Depending upon the state, some nurse practitioners can also write prescriptions.

CERTIFICATION AND REGISTRATION

Certification is recognition that a person has achieved the level of education and skills required to perform the activities of a specific profession. Unlike licensing, certification is usually voluntary. It's also usually granted by a national professional organization rather than by a state government.

Registration involves being placed on a list of people who are considered qualified to engage in a specific profession. Like certification, it's usually voluntary. It's also usually handled by a professional organization. However, some states offer registration for certain allied health professions as well.

Registration is similar to certification in other ways, too.

- Both generally require that certain standards of education and training be met.
- Both usually involve passing an exam on the knowledge and skills the profession requires.
- Because both are often voluntary, neither is usually needed to engage in the profession, as long as the person is qualified otherwise.

ACCREDITATION

To become certified or registered, an allied health professional generally must first complete an accredited education and training program. **Accreditation** is approval given to programs that meet certain specific standards. The two main accrediting organizations in the allied health professions, including medical assisting programs, are:

- the Commission on Accreditation of Allied Health Education Programs (CAAHEP)
- the Accrediting Bureau of Health Education Schools (ABHES)

Certified Medical Assistant Certification

The American Association of Medical Assistants (AAMA) is a professional association that certifies qualified medical assistants as Certified Medical Assistants (CMAs). Here are the requirements:

- completion of a medical assisting program that's accredited by CAAHEP or ABHES
- passing grade on the national CMA exam (It's scored pass/fail only.)
- a clean record with no felony convictions (This requirement can be set aside in certain circumstances, however.)

Membership in AAMA is *not* required for certification. But members pay a lower certification fee than nonmembers do.

Registered Medical Assistant Registration

Registered Medical Assistant (RMA) is a credential offered by the American Medical Technologists (AMT). There are several ways to become an RMA. All require that you be at least 18 years old and have a high school diploma or GED.

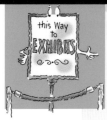

Exhibits

THE HEALTH CARE TEAM

Many kinds of practitioners are needed to provide medical care to patients today. Although the practitioners function as a team, each one is limited to the duties required by her scope of practice.

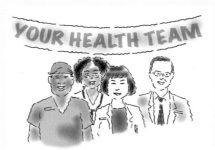

Here are some of the allied health professionals and paraprofessionals you may meet in a medical office, depending on the office's size and the kinds of medicine practiced. Like you, each is responsible for understanding the laws and rules that relate to her job. Many of these jobs require registration or certification by a national organization or by the state.

- *Dietitian*—educates and assists patients with dietary and nutritional needs

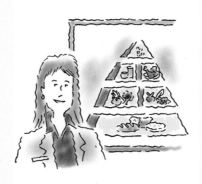

- *ECG technician*—measures and records the heart's electrical activity with an electrocardiogram (ECG) machine
- *EEG technician*—operates electroencephalogram (EEG) equipment to record the electrical activity of the brain
- *Laboratory technician*—performs simple diagnostic tests on blood, urine, and other body fluids and secretions

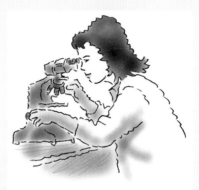

- *Medical transcriptionist*—converts information dictated by the physician into printed material for patients' medical records
- *Phlebotomist*—draws blood from patients for diagnostic testing or other purposes
- *Radiologic technologist*—positions patients for x-rays, operates x-ray equipment, and develops x-ray films for viewing

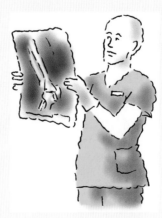

- *Respiratory therapist*—provides breathing tests and treatments to patients
- *Sonographer*—performs ultrasound examinations that provide images of the functioning of internal organs and fetuses

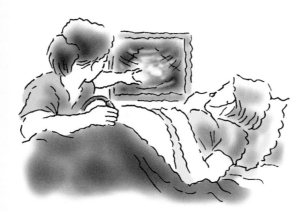

To be registered on the basis of education, you must pass the national RMA exam. You also must complete a medical assisting program that meets one of the following standards:

- accredited by CAAHEP or ABHES
- accredited by another organization that's approved by the U.S. Department of Education
- recognized as a formal medical services training program of the U.S. Army

Interested applicants can also qualify on the basis of experience. Applicants must meet one of the following requirements:

- employment as a medical assistant for at least five years and a passing grade on the national RMA exam
- employment as a medical assistant for at least three of the past five years and a passing grade on another approved medical assisting exam, such as to be a CMA (These applicants do not have to take the RMA exam.)

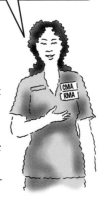

Most states don't require formal training to work as a medical assistant. Being a CMA or RMA shows that you meet national standards of quality.

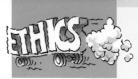

Ethics in Action | WHO AM I?

Many patients think that everyone they see in a lab coat is a physician and every person in a uniform is a nurse. If a patient calls you "nurse," professional ethics require you to correct them with your proper title. Calling *yourself* a nurse, or causing a patient to believe that you're a nurse, is more than unethical—it's illegal. The nurse practice act in most states bars anyone who's not a registered nurse or licensed practical nurse from representing himself as a nurse or using the title "nurse." If a patient mistakenly refers to you as a nurse or other medical professional, take that as an opportunity to explain your job as a medical assistant. This way you can avoid confusion and help patients understand your chosen career!

Medical Practice Acts

About 100 years ago or so, anyone who wanted to call himself a physician could do so. In fact, anyone who wanted to practice medicine could do so. Maybe you've seen western movies in which a barber or the undertaker was also the physician because he had the instruments that were needed. Well, that was true! Some physicians had medical training. But many others had little or none. This made the quality of medical care uncertain at best.

Gradually, trained physicians became tired of untrained physicians tarnishing their good names. Working with other people who wanted safer health care, they convinced state governments to pass laws limiting the practice of medicine to persons who were qualified to do so.

THE STATE IS IN CONTROL

Today, every state has a medical practice act that controls the practice of medicine in that state. It does so in the following ways:

- defines the practice of medicine
- forbids the practice of medicine without a license
- empowers a board of physicians and public members to license physicians and police the profession
- establishes the requirements and methods for issuing licenses

- sets standards for suspending, revoking, and renewing physicians' licenses (To **suspend** something is to temporarily take it away, and to **revoke** it is to take it away permanently.)

All states also have nurse practice acts that control the practice of nursing in the same way. Both the medical practice act and the nurse practice act may have an impact upon those tasks that may be legally delegated to a medical assistant within a particular state.

WHO PRACTICES MEDICINE?

Most medical practice acts define the practice of medicine as diagnosing, treating, or prescribing to cure or prevent any human injury, disease, ailment, deformity, or physical or mental condition. For many years, only physicians were permitted to practice medicine. Today, however, medical boards are allowing new types of health care providers—such as physician assistants and nurse practitioners—to perform some of these tasks.

LICENSE TO HEAL

Obtaining a license to practice medicine is a long, three-step process that involves:

1. meeting an education requirement
2. satisfying a training requirement
3. passing an examination

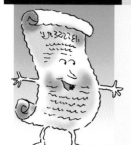

Legal Brief NO LICENSE? NO PROBLEM

There are usually only four situations when the physician is not required to have a license to practice medicine in a state.

- The physician works for the government. For example, the physician may work as an army, navy, or air force physician practicing at a military hospital or on a base, or as an employee of the U.S. Public Health Service.
- The physician is engaged solely in medical research and does not treat patients.
- The physician has recently moved into the state and is in the process of obtaining a license there.
- The physician is providing treatment in an emergency situation.

In addition, to get a license physicians must be:

- at least 21 years old in most states
- of good moral character
- a resident of the state in which they will practice

School Days

To meet the education requirement for a license to practice medicine a person must:

1. graduate from a four-year college or university; most physicians have a degree in one of the biological sciences, although it's not required

2. graduate from an approved four-year medical school; graduates of medical schools outside the United States and Canada must meet additional requirements

Students who graduate from a college of medicine receive a doctor of medicine (MD) degree. Those who graduate from a college of osteopathic medicine earn a doctor of osteopathy (DO) degree. In either case, the person has earned the title "doctor." But she is not yet allowed to practice medicine.

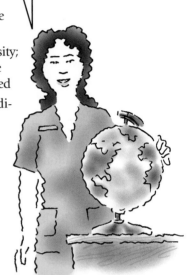

Some students choose to attend medical school outside the United States and Canada. They must meet additional requirements before becoming licensed physicians.

OSTEOPATHY

Osteopathy is a type of medicine that emphasizes treating the "whole person." A doctor of osteopathy looks at the connection between all the body's systems instead of focusing on individual systems or parts.

Of some 635,000 physicians in the United States, about 35,000 are DOs. Twenty-four of the nation's medical schools give DO degrees, compared to 125 that graduate MDs. The education required for each degree is similar.

DOs are licensed to practice medicine in all 50 states. In 14 states, however, the practice of osteopathic medicine is controlled by a different board than the one that licenses MDs.

Training Up

After graduating from medical school, a physician must complete a **residency.** This is a period of hands-on training in treating patients in a hospital. The first year of residency is called an **internship.** During the internship, physicians gain basic experience with various specialties in medicine. Interns rotate among the hospital's various specialties so that they are exposed to all aspects of health care within the hospital. If a physician wants to specialize, he must complete between two and six more years of training in that area of medicine.

Passing the Test

All 50 states require new physicians to pass the United States Medical Licensing Examination (USMLE). This national exam has three parts, or "steps."

1. Step 1 of the USMLE tests knowledge of the sciences involved in the practice of medicine. It's taken while the person is a student in medical school.

2. Step 2 tests if the person can apply her medical knowledge and skills to patient care under supervision. It's usually taken right before or right after graduating from medical school.

3. Step 3 tests the physician's ability to apply her knowledge and skills without supervision. It's usually taken near the end of the physician's internship or after the internship is complete.

Each step must be passed before the next step can be taken. All states require that physicians pass all three steps to be licensed to practice medicine.

Students or graduates of medical schools outside the United States or Canada can take steps 1 and 2 of the USMLE. But they must prove that their school meets U.S. standards to enter a residency program in the United States and take step 3 of the exam.

Board Certified and Approved!

Nearly three-fourths of U.S. physicians are specialists. After completing the additional two- to six-year residency in their specialty, these physicians can become "board certified" in their area of medicine. This requires passing an exam in their medical specialty. About 23 specialties have boards that offer these exams. These boards certify physicians who meet their requirements as "diplomats" or "fellows" in that specialty.

This certification shows a high level of competence in a medical field. It enables the physician to use the term "board certified" in advertising his services. It also allows physicians to use initials like the following in addition to the MD or DO after their names:

- DAPD (Diplomat of the American Board of Pediatrics)
- FACS (Fellow of the American College of Surgeons)
- FACOG (Fellow of the American College of Obstetrics and Gynecology)

ALPHABET SOUP

You'll see a variety of letter combinations after the names of many health care workers. In general, these abbreviations show that the person has achieved a higher-than-average level of training, skill, and knowledge in her profession. The abbreviations CMA and RMA that some medical assistants can use are a good example.

It may be difficult to remember what all the letter combinations mean that follow people's names. But besides the ones you've already seen in this chapter, here are a few more you're likely to come across in a medical office:

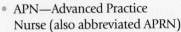

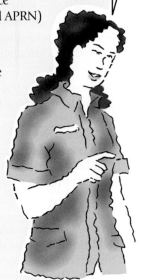

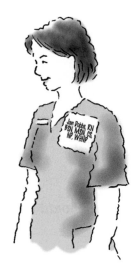

If you get any more credentials, we're going to have to order you a larger name tag.

- APN—Advanced Practice Nurse (also abbreviated APRN)
- CNS—Clinical Nurse Specialist
- CNM—Certified Nurse Midwife
- CRT—Certified X-Ray Technologist
- FNP—Family Nurse Practitioner
- MSN—Master of Science in Nursing (a postgraduate degree)
- WHNP—Women's Health Nurse Practitioner

MOVIN' ON

A physician who's licensed to practice medicine in one state and who moves to another state can usually be licensed in the new state without having to retake the licensing exam. Here's how:

- through reciprocity
- by endorsement

No matter the method applied, the physician's current license must be in good standing and not revoked, suspended, or expired.

In times past, physicians who got into trouble with a medical board sometimes just moved to another state. They would get a new license there and resume practicing medicine. Now, modern technology has made that difficult to do.

When a medical board punishes a physician for misbehavior today, it reports its action to one or more national data banks. A **data bank** is a large amount of information about something that is usually stored on a computer. For example, the Federation Physician Data Center (FPDC) is a data bank run by the Federation of State Medical Boards. The federal government also runs two data banks that track bad behavior in the practice of medicine.

National data banks like the FPDC make it easy to find out if a physician applying for a license has been disciplined in another state. The new state's medical board can then decide whether to deny the application based on this information. Later in this chapter, you'll read about the federal government's data banks and how they're also used to regulate health care.

Reciprocity

Reciprocity is giving advantages or privileges in return for advantages of privileges received. Licensing by reciprocity requires an agreement between two states. An example of reciprocity would be if Ohio's medical board agrees to accept California's licenses as evidence that the physician meets Ohio's licensing requirements. In return, California's medical board agrees to accept Ohio's licenses.

Endorsement

If a physician moves to a state that has no reciprocity agreement with the state where he's currently licensed, his new state board can license him by **endorsement**. This occurs when the new state's medical board judges that his qualifications meet its requirements for a license without having to take a state licensing exam.

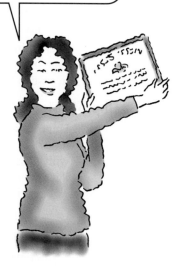

Committing a crime can end a physician's practice of medicine.

DON'T LOSE THAT LICENSE!

A physician's license can be suspended or revoked for several reasons:

- conviction of a felony
- unprofessional conduct
- fraud
- personal or professional incapacity

Professional incompetence, such as negligence or malpractice, can also affect a physician's license, depending on how serious or frequent the acts of incompetence.

A physician whose license has been revoked must give up practicing medicine. If the license is suspended, she can't practice medicine during the period of the suspension.

In general, serious offenses will cause a medical board to revoke a license. Lesser offenses are more likely to result in suspension. Repeated problems eventually may lead to revocation, however.

Revoking or suspending a license is not automatic. If the physician challenges the board's action, a hearing must be held. The physician has the same basic rights as a defendant in a courtroom trial:

- a right to a written description of the charges
- a right to appear before the board and present a defense
- a right to be represented by a lawyer
- a right to present evidence, call witnesses, and question witnesses for the other side
- a right to appeal an unfavorable decision to a court of law

In most cases, the physician can continue to practice until the hearing and appeals process is completed.

Felony Convictions

The following crimes can cost a physician her license:

- rape and other sexual assaults
- Medicare or Medicaid fraud
- violations of drug laws
- tax evasion

These crimes do not have to be committed in the office—or even be related to the practice of medicine—for a physician's license to be revoked.

Unprofessional Conduct

Unprofessional conduct is bad behavior that may not rise to the level of a crime. In some states, the board will charge the physician with gross immorality instead of unprofessional conduct. But even if it's not illegal, it's behavior that's a serious breach of ethics.

Behaviors that are viewed as unprofessional conduct include:

- using unprofessional methods or treatments
- betraying patient confidentiality
- sexual misconduct

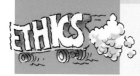

Ethics in Action · FEE SPLITTING

If one physician pays another to refer patients to her, it's called **fee splitting**. Paying for referrals is a serious violation of professional ethics. In some states it's a felony as well. It can also be a federal crime. The penalty for paying or receiving money to refer a patient for treatment paid for by Medicare or Medicaid is five years in prison, a $25,000 fine, or both.

- falsifying records
- fee splitting

Fraud

Fraud is the intentional deceiving of someone in order to receive some kind of gain. Some states include this behavior as part of unprofessional conduct. Examples of fraud include:

- falsifying medical reports
- falsely advertising "miracle cures" or promising them to patients
- falsifying credentials, including a license, qualifications for a license, or an application for a license

Falsely billing patients' health plans for services is also fraud. You'll read about this type of fraud later in this chapter.

Personal or Professional Incapacity

Incapacity is the lack of ability to do something—in this case, the inability to safely engage in the practice of medicine. Personal conditions that may limit a physician's ability to practice medicine include:

- substance abuse, including alcoholism or drug abuse
- senility, mental illness, or other mental incapacity
- other illness or injury (for example, a surgeon losing a finger in an accident)

LICENSE AND CERTIFICATION RENEWAL

Even if a physician stays out of trouble, his license to practice medicine doesn't last forever. It will expire, usually after three to five years, unless he renews it. To do this in most states, he must show that he's completed between 30 and 50 hours (depending on the state) of continuing education. **Continuing education, or CE,** is instruction that keeps people up to date in an area of knowledge or skills.

Continuing education is required of most licensed professionals, from accountants to nurses, to renew their licenses. Renewal of certifications and registrations typically requires continuing education, too.

Continuing Education

Continuing education is usually measured in units called *CEUs,* which stands for *continuing education units.* In general, each hour of instruction is worth one CEU.

Colleges, professional organizations, and companies in the business of providing continuing education provide these opportunities. In the health care industry, hospitals, drug companies, and makers of medical equipment often offer continuing education, too.

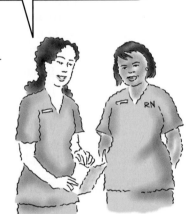

We should both go to this workshop. It's approved for 8 CEUs for nurses and 6 CEUs for certified medical assistants.

State licensing boards and other groups that issue credentials often approve continuing education providers in advance. This means that the provider's continuing education will count for renewal of the credential. If a person takes continuing education from an unapproved provider, that continuing education must be approved on a case-by-case basis. The number of CEUs that it's worth depends on its length and content. For example, an eight-hour program might earn a registered nurse only seven CEUs if one hour isn't relevant to what nurses do.

CONTINUING EDUCATION FOR PHYSICIANS

The continuing education that physicians must obtain is known as continuing medical education, or CME. It usually involves attending:

- seminars and workshops
- sessions at conferences held by professional medical organizations
- credit or noncredit classes offered by educational institutions

A **seminar** is a meeting at which advanced information is discussed. A **workshop** is a meeting that focuses on techniques and skills in a field.

For license renewal, any kind of approved CME is usually okay. But if a physician is board certified, the CME has to be related to her specialty to count toward renewing that credential.

Renewing CMA and RMA Credentials

CMA certification is good for five years. It can be renewed by passing the exam again or by showing evidence of completing 60 CEUs over a five-year period with a required number in each category of administrative, general, and clinical tasks.

The RMA credential is good for three years. Renewal requires 30 hours of continuing education. Work experience and college courses can also be used to meet the requirement if they're related to medical assisting.

Medical Practices and the Law

As you probably realize by now, a great many laws, rules, and regulations affect how medicine is practiced in the United States. You've just read about how the law determines who can practice medicine, and even what practicing medicine means. Later in this chapter, you'll learn about some laws that regulate the financial side of a medical practice. But now, let's look at two laws that shape how medicine is practiced. These laws are:

- Good Samaritan laws
- the Controlled Substances Act

GOOD SAMARITAN LAWS

In most states, the laws that regulate health care include a Good Samaritan Act. (A "good Samaritan" is a person who unselfishly helps others.) **Good Samaritan laws** protect people—including physicians and other health care providers—from being sued for negligence if they help an injured victim in an emergency.

For example, suppose that you're going to lunch, and you come upon someone who's been hit by a car. Your state's Good Samaritan Act does not require you to help the person (except in Vermont). But if you do try to assist, the person usually can't sue you if your aid doesn't help or causes more harm.

There are several limits on this protection, however. Here's what you need to know.

Standard of Care

Emergency care provided under a Good Samaritan Act must meet the reasonable person standard. This standard will be higher for a good Samaritan who has medical training than it will for someone with no medical training. A physician who gives help in an emergency will be held to the highest standard of all.

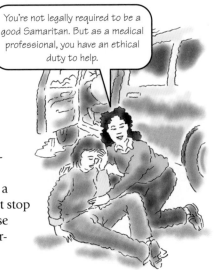

> You're not legally required to be a good Samaritan. But as a medical professional, you have an ethical duty to help.

However, the standard of care a medical professional will be held to is lower than the normal standard of care. That's because it's an emergency situation. It's also because the help is being given in a place where medical equipment and supplies are not available.

Duty of Care

Once a good Samaritan decides to help a victim, she then has a legal duty to keep giving aid until someone more qualified arrives. As a medical assistant, that means you should not stop helping the victim until a physician or a nurse arrives on the scene. It also includes the emergency squad, of course, and the police, once they take over responsibility for the victim.

The Samaritan-Victim Relationship

A good Samaritan should never allow the victim to pay her for her help. That's because accepting payment creates an implied contract between the Samaritan and the victim. If there's a contract and things go bad, the Good Samaritan Act may not apply.

Negligence and Gross Negligence

If you show due care and act in good faith in helping a victim, the Good Samaritan Act can protect you even if your actions cause the victim more harm. There are exceptions, however. You won't be protected it your actions are grossly negligent.

Behaviors that could be viewed as negligent in normal circumstances are often acceptable in emergency situations. However, **gross negligence** is action that was taken so carelessly that the good Samaritan showed little or no concern for the harm he might cause. An example would be treating a victim's sprained wrist while ignoring his heavy bleeding from a severed artery.

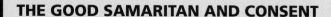

Legal Brief THE GOOD SAMARITAN AND CONSENT

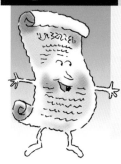

Even in an emergency, you must get the victim's consent for treatment. The only exceptions are if the victim is unconscious or incompetent—that is, unable to function properly. For example, an accident victim might be conscious but unable to respond. Many times, "incompetence" can be a judgment call. But if a victim seems alert and refuses help, you must go along with her wishes.

That would be gross negligence. It also would not meet the requirement of due care. **Due care** is behavior that meets the reasonable person standard.

Gross negligence is almost as bad as deliberately causing harm. Of course, someone who intentionally harms the victim is not protected by good Samaritan laws either. Deliberately harming someone is not acting in good faith, which is another requirement of good Samaritan laws. **Good faith** is a sincere effort to act properly and appropriately.

Emergencies in the Office

Good Samaritan laws don't apply to medical office emergencies. You're not required to give aid outside the office. In the office that's generally not true. If a disoriented person stumbles into the office, for example, and with slurred speech asks for help, you shouldn't just ask him to leave. You might be correct in assuming that he's under the influence of drugs or alcohol. But if it's a stroke instead, he's likely to sue you for not providing emergency care!

CONTROLLED SUBSTANCES LAWS

Each state has laws that limit the sale and use of substances with a high risk for causing dependence and abuse. These items are called **controlled substances.** They range from illegal substances, such as heroin and marijuana, to prescription drugs, such as painkillers.

Controlled substances laws apply to everyone from criminals, who illegally use or sell them, to physicians, who are licensed to use and prescribe many of them in treating patients. Because state laws vary widely, Congress passed a Uniform Controlled Substances Act (UCSA) to create a standard drug policy for the nation.

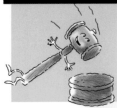

What's the Verdict?

THE GOOD SAMARITAN IN THE COMMUNITY

Your friend asks you to volunteer to provide first aid at a fun run in the community. You're not positive that you're qualified to take on this role; however, your friend says you'll be protected by good Samaritan laws if anything were to go wrong. Is your friend correct?

The Verdict: No, your friend is not right this time! Good Samaritan laws exist to protect health care workers who offer aid in an emergency situation. You can't sign up to provide health care at a fun run or give immunizations at a community health fair and assume that the good Samaritan laws will protect you in case anything goes wrong. If you plan to volunteer at such an event, first check with the organization to find out what laws are protecting you.

The UCSA is commonly called the Controlled Substances Act. A medical practice must pay attention to the requirements of this federal law as well as to its state drug laws. The requirements of some state drug laws may be stricter than the Controlled Substances Act. When this happens, the state requirements must be followed.

Your DEAs Are Numbered!

Each physician who's registered with the DEA receives a DEA registration number. This number must appear on all prescriptions the physician writes for controlled substances.

To get a DEA number, the physician must apply to the DEA and provide the following information:

- the physician's type of business
- the schedules of the drugs the physician is likely to use or prescribe
- the license the physician holds, as well as any state registrations to prescribe controlled substances
- any information about the physician's own use of controlled substances

A physician's DEA number must be renewed every three years. As a medical assistant, you may be responsible for keeping track of this.

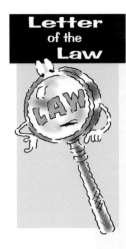

Letter of the Law

THE CONTROLLED SUBSTANCES ACT

Congress passed the Controlled Substances Act in 1970 and renewed it in 1990. It has also been amended, or added to, several times over the years. Here's a summary of the law and how it affects the practice of medicine.

- It divides controlled substances into five groups, called "schedules," based on their potential for abuse.
- Physicians who administer or prescribe these drugs must be registered with the **Drug Enforcement Administration (DEA),** the government agency that enforces the UCSA.
- Controlled substances must be kept locked in a cabinet when not being used. Your office must report any thefts immediately to the nearest DEA office and to the police.
- A record of how controlled substances are used must be made and kept for two years. These records must include the following information:
  1. the name and amount of each drug given to patients
  2. the name of the patient who received the drug
  3. the date the drug was given and why it was given
- You must make a note in a patient's chart each time a controlled substance is given or prescribed.
- You must maintain records of the amount of controlled substances ordered from suppliers for two years.
- Every office must complete an inventory of the supply of controlled substances every two years. The records of the inventory must be kept for two years.

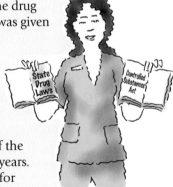

If your state requires keeping drug records longer than the UCSA does, you must obey the stricter state law.

The DEA at the Door!

DEA agents may appear at an office at any time to see if the office is complying with the UCSA. No advance warning is required. The agents will probably want to inspect the records the law requires to be kept. They may compare the office's drug inventory records to the records of drugs ordered from

The Drug Schedules of the Controlled Substances Act		
Schedule	**Drug Class**	**Examples**
I	Drugs with a high potential for abuse and no accepted medical use	Heroin, marijuana, LSD, peyote
II	Drugs with a medical use but high potential for abuse and severe physical or psychological dependence	Opium, morphine, cocaine, codeine, oxycodone, amphetamines, methamphetamines
III	Drugs with a medical use, less potential for abuse than Schedule II drugs, and moderate-to-low physical or psychological dependence	Many barbiturates (a class of pain-killing drugs), codeine with aspirin, or acetaminophen
IV	Drugs containing narcotics (a class of pain killing drugs) in combination with other drugs, with moderate potential for abuse and limited physical or psychological dependence	Mild depressants and stimulants, mild tranquilizers, some antidiarrheals
V	Drugs containing small amounts of narcotics with low potential for abuse and limited physical or psychological dependence	Cough medications with codeine, analgesics, some antidiarrheals

suppliers and those given to patients. A problem will occur if the amount of any drug ordered minus the amount of it given to patients doesn't equal the supply of that drug on hand in the cabinet.

Combating Malpractice and Fraud

In 1986 the federal government began an effort to improve the practice of medicine in the United States. This effort has concentrated on two areas:

- to combat malpractice and the rising number of malpractice suits (You read about malpractice and this trend in Chapters 3 and 4.)
- to combat fraud and the rising cost of health care (It's estimated that as much as $1 of every $10 the nation spends on health care is the result of fraud and abuse in the system.)

The Health Insurance Portability and Accountability Act of 1996 (HIPAA), which you read about in Chapter 3, was part of this effort to improve health care. Among its many reforms, the act streamlined and standardized how insurance claims are

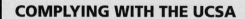

By the Book | COMPLYING WITH THE UCSA

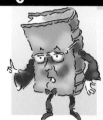

Serious or repeated violations of the Controlled Substances Act can cost a physician his license or shut down a medical office. Here's what you can do to help make sure your office stays in compliance with the UCSA.

- Keep an eye out for any controlled substances left out in the open after being used. Return them to the locked cabinet.

- Also keep an eye out for prescription pads that have been left in a place where patients could get their hands on them. Like controlled substances, blank prescription forms should be kept locked up when they're not being used.

- Be alert to any requests or behavior by patients that suggests they may be deliberately seeking controlled substances from the physician. Report your suspicions to the physician.

  If your medical assisting role includes administrative duties, you may be responsible for maintaining inventories of controlled substances and keeping inventory records.

  Also, it's a good idea to order prescription pads that have sequentially numbered forms, much like checks in a checkbook. Numbering blank prescription forms helps keep track of them and makes missing or stolen forms easier to detect.

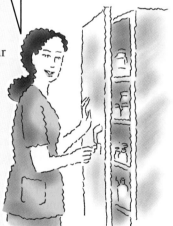

Keep controlled substances and prescription pads locked up when they're not being used.

filed. In part, this change was to help combat fraud and abuse in billing patients' health care plans. In medical billing, **fraud** is billing for services that were not provided, and **abuse** is billing for services that were provided but which were not needed.

THE HEALTHCARE INTEGRITY AND PROTECTION DATA BANK

Another way that HIPAA fought fraud was by creating the Healthcare Integrity and Protection Data Bank (HIPDB). This is a national program to collect and report information about billing fraud and abuse.

> Health plans and government agencies report to HIPDB the names of providers—such as medical offices, hospitals, and medical supply companies—they've taken action against for fraud or abuse. Other health plans and government agencies can then get this information. It's not available to the general public, however.

But even before HIPAA, two events in 1986 launched the government's effort to reform the health care system:

- passage of the Health Care Quality Improvement Act
- changes in the False Claims Act that encouraged citizens to sue providers who were committing fraud against the U.S. government

THE HEALTH CARE QUALITY IMPROVEMENT ACT

The Health Care Quality Improvement Act (HCQIA) strengthened peer review as a method of maintaining high standards in medical practice. **Peer review** is a process in which a committee of physicians judges the charges of a physician's wrongdoing. HCQIA strengthened peer review by protecting members of these committees from being sued by the accused physician if she doesn't agree with their findings.

Among the most important reforms of HCQIA was its creation of the National Practitioner Data Bank (NPDB). The law requires that payments in malpractice suits and actions against a physician's license or professional memberships must be reported to the NPDB. Hospitals that revoke a physician's privileges to admit and treat patients must report this action to the NPDB as well.

Hospitals must also check with the NPDB for reports on a physician before granting him privileges to practice there. To renew privileges, hospitals must also check every two years on physicians who already have privileges.

THE FALSE CLAIMS ACT

The False Claims Act (FCA) is an old law. Congress passed it in the 1860s to stop dishonest suppliers of goods to the Union Army during the American Civil War. The law remained on the books after the war ended. It continued to be used mainly to target defense contractors who were overcharging the U.S. military.

Since the 1990s, however, most of the cases brought under the FCA have been for fraud against the government's medical and health insurance programs. The three main programs are:

- **Medicare,** the government's health insurance program for retired persons, aged 65 and over
- **Medicaid,** the government's health insurance program that pays the costs of medical care for low-income individuals
- **Tri-Care,** the government's health insurance program for military families; until fairly recently, it was called CHAMPUS

Today, the FCA is sometimes called the "whistleblower law." (A **whistleblower** is someone who exposes wrongdoing even though she hasn't been harmed.) That's because the law allows anyone who becomes aware of false claims made to the federal government to sue on the government's behalf. The whistleblower gets a share of the money that's recovered as a result.

During the American Civil War, the government was too busy fighting the war to investigate and prosecute fraud itself. So it depended on private citizens to do so. Today, the government is so big and has so many programs, that it continues to "pay" informers to expose misuse of the taxpayers' money.

Whistleblowers have filed more than 4,000 lawsuits under the False Claims Act since 1986. The government has recovered more than $6 billion as a result. Of this amount, more than $960 million has been paid to the whistleblowers.

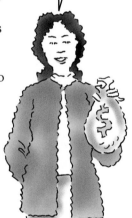

> Money is always nice, of course, but ethics require you to report wrongdoing, even if there's no reward.

Legal Brief   *QUI TAM*

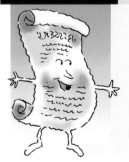

The whistleblower provisions of the False Claims Act depend on a common law principle known as *qui tam.* This Latin term is short for a longer phrase that means "he who sues for the king sues for himself."

Generally, only the first person to file a *qui tam* lawsuit is rewarded. Also, if one person uncovers the fraud, but a second person files the suit, only the second person is entitled to a share of the money that's recovered.

Legal Brief   CONSPIRACY TO COMMIT FRAUD

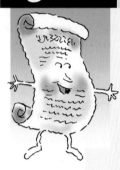

Medical assistants are routinely asked to prepare claims to be submitted to a patient's health plan. A medical assistant who agrees to file a claim that does not accurately reflect the actual situation could be found guilty of conspiracy to commit fraud. **Conspiracy** is cooperating with someone to ignore or disobey the law.

For example, suppose a physician asks you to put a false diagnosis on a claim form, so the patient's health plan will pay for a treatment the physician has given. The physician is committing fraud. By filling out the form as he asks, you're participating in the fraud. That makes you part of a criminal conspiracy.

TYPES OF MEDICAL FRAUD

There are three basic types of medical fraud. Most of the practices in these areas are illegal under state law as well as federal law. They include:

- procedures fraud involves providing treatments that are not needed
- kickbacks involves profiting from the referral of patients
- billing fraud (the most common type of medical fraud)

Procedures Fraud

Providing a treatment that a patient doesn't need is both unethical and illegal. Then billing the patient or the patient's health plan for that unneeded procedure is a separate, second act of fraud.

Medicare and some health plans also have rules about who provides some treatments. For example, they may require that a licensed professional perform certain procedures in order to pay for them, even if the state's medical practice act allows others to do so. Always be careful when billing in order to avoid fraud.

Kickbacks and Referrals

A **kickback** is a payment made to someone in order to obtain her business. Paying or accepting money for patient referrals is illegal under state and federal laws. If the referral involves treatments or products that would be paid for by Medicare or Medicaid, it's also a violation of the Medicare-Medicaid Antifraud and Abuse Amendments of 1977.

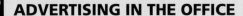

What's the Verdict? ADVERTISING IN THE OFFICE

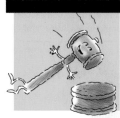

A sales person visits a medical office and wants to leave brochures in the patient waiting room that advertise the services of a nearby weight-loss clinic. The office manager thinks this is a good idea, but the medical assistant isn't so sure. Should the sales person be allowed to leave the brochures?

The Verdict: Medical office waiting rooms frequently contain pamphlets that promote medical products or services. Such materials don't violate anti-kickback laws as long as the office accepts no money or other favors in return. But even though it's legal, the ethics of it may be another matter. The medical assistant was right to question this literature, especially if it promises unrealistic results. Some patients may assume that products or services advertised in waiting room brochures have the physicians' recommendation. For this reason, such brochures should be carefully screened. Only literature the physicians are comfortable with should be displayed.

Referring patients to any facility, such as a hospital or a lab, which is fully or partly owned by the referring physician, is illegal. The Ethics in Patient Referral Act of 1989 bans such referrals if they'll be paid for by Medicare or Medicaid. But regardless of who pays, these referrals also violate other federal and state laws.

Billing Fraud

Many billing frauds involve improper use of diagnosis codes (ICD) or current procedural terminology (CPT) codes. Diagnosis codes tell a patient's health plan why the patient saw the physician. CPT codes tell the health plan what services were provided. In general, the services provided must be called for by the patient's diagnosis. If they're not appropriate for the diagnosis, the health plan usually won't pay for the services.

Here are some coding practices that are illegal:

- **upcoding**—billing for complex services when only simple services were performed; billing for brand-name drugs when generic drugs were provided; or listing treatment for a more complicated diagnosis than was the case
- **unbundling**—using two or more CPT codes to bill tests or services separately in order to obtain a higher payment,

when one code would cover a group of tests or services provided

Other billing practices considered to be fraud are:

- billing for services that were never performed (called **phantom billing**)
- charging for equipment or supplies that were never ordered
- billing for new or expensive equipment but providing the patient with used or cheaper equipment instead
- routinely forgiving patients' copayments (a **copayment** is a small sum of money some health plans require the patient to pay as part of the insurance contract), which could be viewed as a breach of contract
- billing for services provided by unqualified or unlicensed workers
- failing to refund overpayments made by patients or their health plans

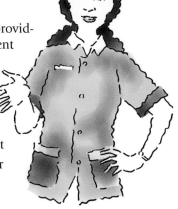

Certain acts that may seem to "help" patients, such as forgiving copayments, are actually considered billing fraud. It's better to follow the letter of the law every time!

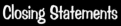
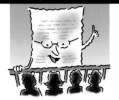

Closing Statements

- States require that physicians and nurses be licensed in order to practice medicine. Professional organizations certify or register other health care workers who meet the standards established for their profession.
- Because medical assistants do not receive the same level of training that nurses receive, it's unlawful for medical assistants to call themselves nurses.
- Each state has a medical practice act that defines the practice of medicine and sets the requirements for obtaining a license to practice it. A state medical board of physicians and members of the public enforces its medical practice act and licenses physicians.
- To obtain a license to practice medicine, a physician must meet an education requirement, complete a residency, and pass a test. Licenses must be renewed every few years by completing a continuing education requirement.
- Licensed physicians who move to another state are usually licensed to practice in that state through reciprocity or endorsement.

- Physicians who engage in wrongdoing can have their licenses suspended or revoked.

- Good Samaritan laws protect health care providers who aid victims in emergencies from being sued if their aid does not help or causes further harm. To get this protection, good Samaritans must act in good faith, show due care, and not be grossly negligent. Good Samaritan laws do not apply to emergencies that occur in a medical office.

- The Controlled Substances Act regulates how medical offices handle and use drugs that have a potential for addiction and abuse. The Drug Enforcement Administration (DEA) enforces the Controlled Substances Act.

- Physicians who administer or prescribe controlled substances must register with the DEA and obtain a DEA number that must appear on all prescriptions for controlled substances.

- Federal and state laws ban fraud and abuse in the practice of medicine. Most medical fraud involves providing treatment that's not needed, profiting from referrals of patients, and illegal practices in billing patients' insurance.

- Federal laws such as the False Claims Act are aimed at fraud and abuse in the federal government's Medicare, Medicaid, and Tri-Care health insurance systems.

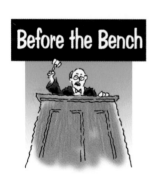

Before the Bench

Answer the following multiple-choice questions.

1. How are licenses, certification, and registration alike?
   a. They are required to practice a profession.
   b. They are all issued by professional organizations.
   c. They usually require passing an examination.
   d. all of the above

2. Medical assistants should *not* call themselves nurses because:
   a. they do not have nursing licenses.
   b. it's unethical to do so.
   c. it's illegal to do so.
   d. all of the above

3. A state's medical practice act:
   a. limits who can engage in the practice of medicine.
   b. licenses registered nurses and nurse practitioners.
   c. registers and certifies allied health professionals.
   d. all of the above

4. Which of the following is *not* a requirement to be licensed to practice medicine?
   a. graduating from an approved medical school
   b. obtaining certification in a medical specialty
   c. completing a training period in a hospital
   d. passing a national examination

5. A physician's license to practice medicine may be suspended or revoked if the physician:
   a. is convicted of a felony.
   b. behaves unprofessionally.
   c. becomes physically incapacitated.
   d. all of the above

6. Which of the following is an example of continuing education?
   a. attending a session at a professional conference
   b. obtaining a license to practice medicine
   c. becoming certified to practice a profession
   d. all of the above

7. Which of the following is true of Good Samaritan laws?
   a. They require health care workers to stop and give aid.
   b. They protect emergency caregivers from lawsuits.
   c. They also apply to emergencies in medical offices.
   d. They protect all behaviors during an emergency.

8. Which of the following is *not* required by the Controlled Substances Act?
   a. numbering the blank forms on a prescription pad
   b. registering physicians who prescribe controlled substances with the DEA
   c. keeping records of controlled substances prescribed
   d. keeping records of controlled substances used

9. Which law is *not* aimed at stopping fraud and abuse in the health care system?
   a. the Ethics in Patient Referral Act
   b. the Health Insurance Portability and Accountability Act
   c. the Health Care Quality Improvement Act
   d. the False Claims Act

10. Which of the following is a type of billing fraud?
   a. upcoding
   b. unbundling
   c. phantom billing
   d. all of the above

Chapter 6

BUILDING HEALTHY PHYSICIAN-PATIENT RELATIONSHIPS

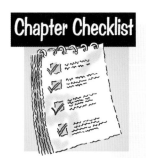

Chapter Checklist

- Summarize the rights and responsibilities of both the physician and the patient

- Explain the differences between an HMO, a PPO, and a POS

- Distinguish between expressed and implied consent and provide examples of both

- List the reasons a minor can obtain medical treatment without a parent's consent

- Discuss the similarities and differences between privacy, confidentiality, and privileged communication

- Identify the types of abuse that must be reported

- Cite four examples of reportable conditions and explain the process of reporting

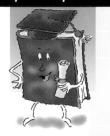

Chapter Competencies

- Identify and respond to issues of confidentiality (CAAHEP 3.c.2.a.)

- Perform within legal and ethical boundaries (CAAHEP 3.c.2.b.)

- Demonstrate knowledge of federal and state health care legislation and regulations (CAAHEP 3.c.2.f.)

- Maintain confidentiality at all times (ABHES 1.b.)

- Use appropriate guidelines when releasing records or information (ABHES 5.c.)

As you've already learned, great changes have occurred in the practice of medicine over time. Not only have group practices replaced the family physician, but the pricing structure has changed as well. In the past, physicians charged patients according to their own fee schedules. Fees are now largely set and paid by health care plans, some of which also influence decisions about the care patients receive. In this chapter, you'll read about the physician-patient relationship and the ways trends have affected it. Change will continue to happen as time goes on. Health care and its delivery are hot topics right now, and you can expect that they will continue to receive a lot of attention. These changes keep things interesting in the medical office. Just because that's the way we've always done it doesn't mean that's the way we'll continue to do it!

And although change is inevitable over time, there are many things that have stayed the same when it comes to the medical office. You'll also learn about aspects of the physician-patient relationship that remain unchanged.

Rights and Responsibilities

Each patient who comes through the medical office door enters with certain basic rights. In addition, the physician has certain responsibilities to all patients that she treats. Finally, physicians have rights, and patients have responsibilities in the physician-patient relationship, too.

PATIENT RIGHTS

Congress has made several attempts to establish federal laws that protect patients' rights, but most have failed to become laws. However, in 1998 the President's Advisory Commission on Consumer Protection and Quality in the Health Care Industry issued a Consumer Bill of Rights and Responsibilities. Many health care organizations and insurance plans have adopted its principles. The Consumer Bill of Rights and Responsibilities outlines patient rights in seven areas:

- information disclosure
- choice of providers and plans
- access to emergency services
- participation in treatment decisions
- respect and nondiscrimination
- confidentiality of health information
- complaints and appeals

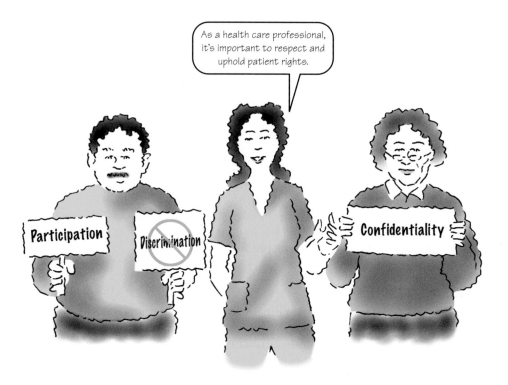

As a health care professional, it's important to respect and uphold patient rights.

Participation

Discrimination

Confidentiality

The spread of managed care has affected rights in several of these areas. **Managed care** is a system that involves the patient's health plan, the physician, and the patient in deciding what treatment the patient should receive, and what the physician will be paid for those services. You'll read more about managed care later in this chapter.

Information Disclosure

Patients have the right to clear and accurate information about their health plan, health care professionals, and health care facilities. If the patient speaks another language or has a physical or mental disability, the patient has a right to assistance so that he can make informed health care decisions.

Many health care plans and providers make pamphlets available to patients that explain their services. Medical offices in areas with large non-English-speaking populations should offer their pamphlets in languages common to the area. At least some staff members should also speak languages common to the neighborhood. (If you speak a second language, be sure to include that information on your resume. The ability to speak another language may be a determining factor when you're being considered for employment.)

Offices should also have a list of translators they may contact if one is required. If an office doesn't have an existing list, most hospitals have a list of translators in the area. Gestures may not suffice when it comes to obtaining a patient's informed consent. How can the patient understand what his rights are if he doesn't understand the language used to explain the procedure or treatment?

Choice of Providers and Plans

Patients have the right to a choice of a variety of high-quality health care providers to meet their personal needs. Some people believe that managed care plans limit this right by requiring that the physician obtain the plan's approval to perform certain procedures or to refer the patient to a specialist. That's why many times the referring physician is called the **gatekeeper.**

Access to Emergency Services

If severe pain, an injury, or sudden illness convinces someone that her health is in serious jeopardy, she has the right to receive emergency services whenever and wherever needed, without prior authorization or financial penalty. However, some managed care plans impose financial penalties on emergency room visits unless these visits result in the patient being admitted to the hospital. Another problem is that the signs and symptoms of many serious illnesses mimic other illnesses and ailments that aren't as severe. A classic example is that a patient may have a crushing feeling in her chest combined with heartburn. This could be something as severe as a heart attack or as simple as indigestion. The problem is that the patient may not know the difference until she's gone to the emergency room. Unfortunately, if the patient is diagnosed with indigestion, the insurance company may not pay for her visit or the many tests that might have been run.

Participation in Treatment Decisions

Patients have the right to know their treatment options and to participate in decisions about their care. Parents, guardians, family members, or other individuals whom they name can represent them if they can't make their own decisions.

This also means that patients have the right to refuse treatment. For example, members of some religious groups oppose certain treatments on religious grounds. On the other hand, physicians have the right to not treat patients whose wishes endanger the prospects for a good outcome.

Respect and Nondiscrimination

Patients have a right to considerate, respectful, and nondiscriminatory care from their physicians, health plan representatives, and other health care providers. In part, this means that physicians can't refuse to treat a patient with AIDS, for example, merely because the patient is HIV positive.

Confidentiality of Health Information

Patients have the right to talk in confidence with health care providers and to have their health care information protected. They also have the right to review and copy their medical record and to request that their physician change their record if it isn't accurate or complete.

However, keep in mind that you never want to leave a patient alone with his original medical record because the record will be the physician's defense if a lawsuit were to occur. If a patient tears a page (or pages) out of his chart, how will the physicians defend themselves? The old saying "If it's not charted, it didn't happen" might prevail here.

Complaints and Appeals

Patients have the right to a fair, fast, and objective review of any complaint they have against their health plan, physicians, hospitals, or other health care personnel. This includes complaints about waiting times, operating hours, the conduct of health care personnel, and the adequacy of health care facilities.

PATIENTS HAVE RESPONSIBILITIES, TOO

The physician-patient relationship isn't all about patients' rights. Patients have certain responsibilities in the relationship, too. These responsibilities include honesty, cooperation, and payment.

Honesty in Communication

Patients must be honest when talking with the physician. This includes providing all information that might be relevant to the patient's condition, diagnosis, and treatment. It means that patients shouldn't withhold information because it might be embarrassing. Incomplete information can lead to an incorrect diagnosis.

Cooperation with the Physician

Patients must cooperate with the physician and follow the physician's instructions. This includes filling all prescriptions and taking all drugs the physician prescribes, as well as following all other orders for treatment after the patient leaves the physician's office. The patient's failure to do this can release a physician from legal responsibility for poor treatment outcomes.

Payment of Fees

Patients must pay the physician's fees for treatment provided. This also means cooperating with the physician's office to obtain payment from the patient's health insurance plan.

THE PHYSICIAN'S RIGHTS AND RESPONSIBILITIES

Physicians have the right to choose the type of medicine they will practice, whether or not they will specialize, and the hours during which they will provide care. Within certain limits, they also have the right to decide how their services will be provided. For example, will the physician give the patient an injection, or will he assign the office nurse or medical assistant to do it?

As a cardiologist, I can't tend to your broken leg. But I'm happy to refer you to a surgeon who can help.

Choosing Patients

Physicians also have the right to choose which patients they will treat. This right has some limits, however. For example, it's appropriate for a *dermatologist* (a physician who specializes in treating skin conditions) to refuse a patient who comes to her with heart disease. In fact, it would be unethical for her to treat this condition.

But a physician can't refuse to treat a patient because of the patient's race, religion, or some other basis that applies to an entire class of people. To do so is discrimination, and discrimination is a violation of a patient's civil rights and of federal law.

PROFESSIONAL COURTESY

Professional courtesy is the practice of treating health care professionals free of charge or for a reduced fee. It's a long-time tradition in the medical profession. However, physicians are not ethically required to extend professional courtesy to other health care providers, or even to accept them as patients.

When to Say Good-Bye

Once a physician accepts a patient for treatment, he has a duty to continue the care, except under certain conditions. These can include the following.

- The patient no longer needs the service—for example, his disease is cured.

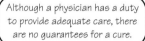

Although a physician has a duty to provide adequate care, there are no guarantees for a cure.

- The patient seeks treatment from another physician, or the physician refers the patient to another physician.

- The patient misses appointments, does not follow the physician's instructions, or in other ways fails to be responsible for his care.

- The patient does not pay his bill or make acceptable arrangements to pay it.

When ending the physician-patient relationship, the physician must be careful to avoid abandoning the patient. You read about abandonment and how to avoid it in Chapter 2.

The practice of medicine also involves other legal and ethical responsibilities and duties. You've read about many of these in earlier chapters—for example, the physician's duty to provide an acceptable standard of care. You'll learn about more physician responsibilities in Chapter 8, when you read about medical codes of ethics.

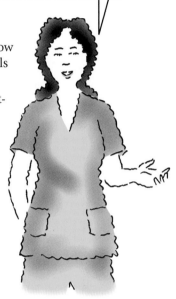

Rights, Responsibilities, and Managed Care

The practice of medicine traditionally involved the physician making treatment decisions with the patient's consent. The physician then billed the patient or the patient's health insurance plan for the treatment that was provided. This traditional system of providing care is known as **fee-for-service.**

However, the high costs of health care have changed the way that medicine is practiced in the United States. One result has been a rapid growth in managed-care organizations since the 1980s.

There are two basic types of managed-care organizations: health maintenance organizations and preferred provider organizations. In general, managed care organizations try to control the costs of health care by limiting the following:

- the patient's choice of physician
- the tests and treatments a physician can order

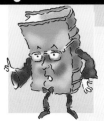

By the Book

WHEN PATIENTS NO LONGER NEED SERVICES

In Chapter 2 you read about the termination letter a medical office must send when a physician no longer wants to treat a patient. But what, if anything, should be done when the patient no longer needs treatment?

Ending the physician-patient relationship because the patient is "cured" is not abandonment. Therefore, a formal termination letter isn't necessary. However, to avoid potential problems in this area, many offices send the patient a letter anyway. It's not a termination letter, but merely a friendly note thanking the patient for the opportunity to serve her. Many surgeons' offices do this because once the surgery is performed, the patient's care is transferred back to the referring physician. The surgeon typically does not need to monitor the patient after the post-op visit.

The letter also advises the patient to call if the problem arises again or if some other service is needed. Such letters are not only a good idea from a legal standpoint, they're also excellent customer service tools.

- second opinions for diagnosis and treatment
- the drugs that can be prescribed
- referrals to specialists and the choice of specialists
- the choice of hospitals and how long a patient can be hospitalized
- the fees that health care providers are paid for their services

HEALTH MAINTENANCE ORGANIZATIONS

Health maintenance organizations (HMOs) are managed-care plans in which physicians treat plan members for a preset payment typically referred to as "prospective payment." Each member chooses a participating physician as his **primary care physician** (PCP). The member must go to the PCP for all care. Referrals for outside tests or treatment by specialists must be made by the patient's PCP, or the plan will not pay for them.

Because the PCP controls the patient's care, this physician is often called the gatekeeper. Many plans further control patient care by requiring the gatekeeper to get approval from the HMO before making such referrals.

In some HMOs each physician receives a yearly payment, called a **capitation payment,** for the members who choose him as PCP. With this type of arrangement, the PCP receives payment whether he sees the patient or not. To make money from this arrangement, a medical practice must keep the total cost of treating these patients lower than the capitation payment it receives for their care.

In other HMOs, the physicians are actual employees of the HMO. In this case, the fixed payment is their annual salary. These physicians also usually receive a bonus based on the HMO's profits for the year. The purpose of this bonus is to encourage the physicians to keep the costs of patient care low by minimizing the tests and procedures ordered.

PREFERRED PROVIDER ORGANIZATIONS

Preferred provider organizations (PPOs) are health plans in which patients are encouraged to use certain providers who have agreed to offer services for reduced fees. The physicians, hospitals, and other providers who are part of a PPO are called **participating providers,** or in-network providers.

"In network" means that the provider is part of the group of providers who've agreed to accept the PPO's reduced fees instead of what they normally charge. In a sense, the PPO and its members get a discount on the physician's normal fees.

PPOs differ from HMOs in three ways.

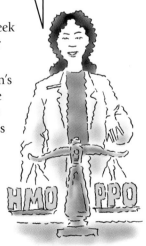

Although HMOs and PPOs are both types of managed-care programs, they each have their own positive and negative features.

- PPOs are fee-for-service plans. Instead of being paid a fixed amount per patient, providers are paid for each service they provide. However, they are paid at a reduced fee.

- There are no gatekeeper physicians. A patient can seek treatment directly from specialists, according to her needs. She is not required to choose a PCP.

- Patients are not forced to seek treatment from the plan's providers. However, going to a provider who's outside the PPO's network requires them to pay a larger share of the costs of their treatment. This penalty encourages plan members to use in-network providers.

Like HMOs, many PPOs require that certain tests and treatments be pre-approved by the plan in order for the plan to pay for them. This exposes them to many of the criticisms often leveled against HMO plans. These criticisms generally involve quality of care, patients' rights, and physicians' legal and ethical responsibilities.

Ethics in Action | THE ETHICS OF MANAGED CARE

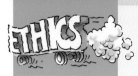

Managed-care plans are designed to reduce the costs of health care. Supporters claim that managed care delivers health care more efficiently. Critics claim that it also affects the care provided. They argue that restricting the physician's freedom to treat patients:

- reduces the quality of medical care
- weakens the physician-patient relationship
- undermines patients' rights and well-being

Managed care can create serious dilemmas for health care providers. Physicians may be unable to do what's best for the patient without risking financial losses or the irritation of plan managers. In fact, physicians who are unwilling or unable to stay within a plan's limits on costs of care may find themselves removed as plan providers. However, skimping on tests and treatments to save money can also expose the physician to charges of negligence and malpractice.

OTHER FORMS OF MANAGED CARE

Although HMOs and PPOs are the most common forms of managed care, other kinds of managed-care systems exist.

Independent Practice Associations

An independent practice association (IPA) is a group of physicians, hospitals, and other providers contracted with an HMO to provide services to the HMO's members. IPAs often provide care for several HMOs.

Point-of-Service Plans

A point-of-service plan (POS) allows members to see other physicians than their PCP, without referral from the PCP. However, they pay a higher share of their cost of care.

Exclusive Provider Organizations

The exclusive provider organization (EPO) is a form of managed care that combines the HMO and PPO systems. Like an HMO, the member's choice of providers is limited to a small group. But like a PPO, providers are paid on a reduced fee-for-service basis.

Physician-Hospital Organizations

A physician-hospital organization is a group of physicians, hospitals, nursing homes, labs, and other providers that work together. They contract with HMOs, insurance plans, or directly with employers to provide services.

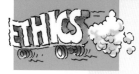

Ethics in Action   TELEMEDICINE

Telemedicine is another form of patient care that takes place by phone or closed-circuit TV and, in recent years, over the Internet. It originally arose because of the need to treat patients in remote areas who didn't have ready access to a physician.

Today telemedicine delivers information and, sometimes, health care between physicians and patients regardless of location. For example, many Internet sites offer patients detailed information from physicians about medical conditions.

The Internet also allows diagnostic tests such as x-rays, CT scans, and ultrasound images to be transmitted from the location where they're performed to be interpreted by physicians in other locations. Closed-circuit TV and real-time computer video allows physicians to examine patients and sometimes even to perform procedures by computerized remote control.

These advances have raised many legal and ethical questions that are related to the physician-patient relationship.

- How can private patient information be protected on the Internet?

- How should physicians who provide telemedicine services be reimbursed?

- How can those who receive information and care via the Internet be assured that the provider is properly credentialed?

- Who should license providers who perform services across state lines— for instance, if the patient lives in one state and the physician practices in another?

States and the federal government have begun passing laws in recent years to deal with these and other telemedicine issues.

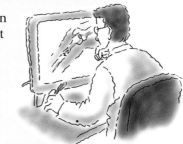

As technological advances continue to change health care, the government will need to create more laws to regulate telemedicine.

Contracts and the Medical Office

You first read about contracts in Chapter 2. You learned that the physician-patient relationship is a contract, even if there's nothing actually in writing. The physician agrees to treat the patient and to provide an acceptable standard of care. In return, the patient agrees to cooperate with and pay for that care. If either party fails to live up to the agreement, the contract is broken or breached. (You also read about breach of contract in Chapter 2.)

- The physician can breach the contract by failing in his duty to provide a proper standard of care—through negligence or malpractice—or by abandoning the patient. In either case, the patient has grounds to sue the physician.

- The patient can breach the contract by not cooperating with his care or by not paying for it. As you read earlier in this chapter, the physician has the right to stop treating the patient under these circumstances.

THREE-PARTY CONTRACTS

Another type of contract that affects the physician-patient relationship is the third-party contract, which you first read about in Chapter 2. In the medical setting, the three parties to this contract are the physician, the patient, and the patient's health insurance plan.

In a sense, this contract is actually three two-party contracts:

- the physician's contract with the patient to provide care
- the patient's contract, or health insurance policy with her insurance plan to pay the costs of the physician's care
- the physician's contract with the insurance company

The contracts together form a three-party contract. See the *Exhibits* feature on page 145.

CONTRACTS AND MANAGED CARE

Medical contracts have been affected by the growth of managed care. Three-party contracts don't exist when the patient's health plan is an HMO. That's because, except for the patient's copayment, the HMO has already paid the physician in advance for the costs of the patient's care. PPOs affect three-party contracts as well.

Three-Party Contracts and PPOs

As you've read, participating providers in PPOs are required to accept a payment for their services that's less than what they charge their other patients. Physicians may still bill patients for balances remaining after the PPO payment, if the patient has copayments and other amounts the plan requires him to pay. However, the balance the patient is responsible for is not based on the physician's full charge for the service. Instead, it must be based on the PPO's discounted rate (also known as the "allowable fee").

For example, suppose the physician charges $100 for a service, but the PPO allows only $80 for that service. If the PPO pays $65, the patient is responsible for $15—the difference between the PPO's allowed rate and its payment. The physician can't bill the patient for the additional $20 difference between the PPO's rate and his full charge.

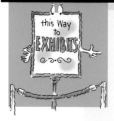

Exhibits   HOW A THREE-PARTY CONTRACT WORKS

1. An insurance company agrees to pay certain costs of a patient's medical care. The terms and limits of this coverage are stated in the health insurance policy, which is a contract between the company and the patient. In return, the patient pays a monthly fee, or "premium," to the insurance company.

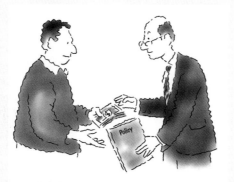

2. The physician bills the insurance company for the costs of the patient's care. The insurance company pays the physician according to the terms of the company's policy (contract) with the patient.

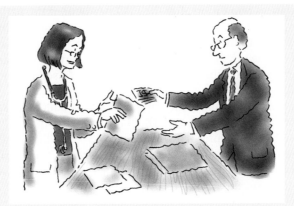

3. The physician then bills the patient for any money that remains outstanding after the insurance company has paid.

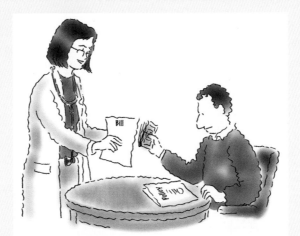

Because third-party contracts aren't enforceable unless they're in writing, many medical offices require patients to sign an agreement before treatment begins that they will pay their bill if their insurance does not. For example, an office may require that a patient sign such an agreement before having an elective procedure. **Elective procedures** are treatments the patient wants but which the insurance company doesn't consider medically necessary. For instance, most cosmetic surgeries—such as liposuction and face-lifts—are elective procedures for which insurance plans usually won't pay.

Other Managed-Care Contracts

A physician must accept the PPO's rate for a service as full payment because of the physician's contract with the PPO. All participating providers sign contracts with the PPO in which they agree to go along with all the plan's rules and regulations, including those regarding fees, referrals, and pre-approval for certain tests and procedures.

In return for agreeing to these conditions, the physician benefits from the PPO's large number of members as potential patients for her practice. Most physicians participate in many PPOs. In fact, because managed care has become so common, a large portion of most physicians' practices are members of PPOs.

Physicians also sign contracts with HMOs. In some cases, the physician agrees to treat only the HMO's patients. In others, she may treat non-HMO patients or the patients of other HMOs as well. It all depends on the terms of the contract. However, like network providers for PPOs, HMO physicians agree to follow procedures designed to keep the costs of health care low.

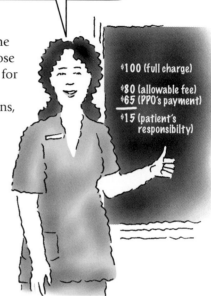

If the patient is a member of a PPO, the amount he owes is based on the PPO's allowable fee, not the physician's full-charge price.

$100 (full charge)

$80 (allowable fee)
$65 (PPO's payment)

$15 (patient's responsibilty)

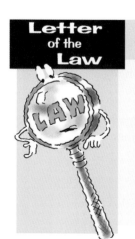

Letter of the Law

THE HMO ACT OF 1973

Congress passed the Health Maintenance Organization Act in 1973 to encourage the growth of managed care in the U.S. health care industry. The law requires that physicians who are part of HMOs devote at least one-third of their time to seeing HMO patients. The law also required companies with more than 25 employees to offer an HMO plan in addition to a traditional group insurance plan. However, that requirement was repealed in 1993.

The Physician-Patient Relationship and Consent

Consent is another topic you've read about in earlier chapters. It's at the heart of the physician-patient relationship. It's also an important part of patients' rights and a physician's responsibilities.

In most cases, a patient can't take part in treatment decisions (a basic patient right) unless he is given the opportunity to consent to them. And the patient can't make good choices about his treatment unless his consent is an informed consent. This means the physician has a responsibility to explain honestly to the patient:

- the advantages and risks of the treatment
- the treatment's possible outcomes
- alternative treatments that are available
- what might happen if the patient refuses the treatment

IMPLIED CONSENT

Not all situations require the patient's informed consent. Routine procedures fall into this category. For example, you don't need to explain the benefits and risks of blood tests to a patient before drawing his blood. Consent occurs when the patient shows by his behavior that he agrees to the procedure. In this example, he might take a seat in the lab chair and roll up his sleeve to expose a vein. Consent that's indicated by a patient's actions is called **implied consent.**

EXPRESSED CONSENT

There are other times, however, when not only is informed consent required, but the patient should sign a form stating that the risks, benefits, and alternatives to the treatment have been explained to him. This type of informed consent is called **expressed consent.** Typically, an expressed consent form will be signed by the physician, the patient, and a witness (usually the medical assistant). The signed form should then be placed in the patient's medical record.

A consent form should be signed any time there's more than a slight risk of harm to the patient. Examples of procedures that require a signed consent form include the following:

- minor office surgery
- radiation therapy
- chemotherapy
- experimental procedures

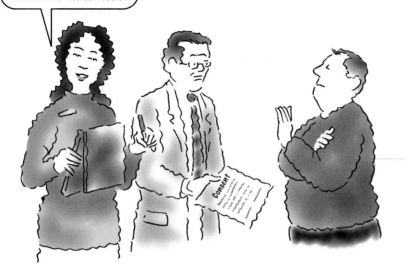

If a patient refuses to sign a consent form, the treatment should not be given. The patient's refusal should be noted in his medical record.

Confidentiality and Patients' Rights

As you've already learned, the privacy of a patient's medical information is among the most sacred of patient rights. Like consent, confidentiality is a central part of the physician-patient relationship. Patients will be less likely to share information such as sexual history, drug use, abortions, and other information that might affect their diagnosis and treatment if such information is not kept confidential. In today's computerized information age, patient privacy has become a major legal and ethical issue and concern.

PRIVILEGED COMMUNICATION

Physicians and all other health care professionals have a legal and ethical responsibility to safeguard patients' privacy by keeping their medical information confidential. The relationship between physician and patient has the same legal protections as the relationship between an attorney and her client.

Like attorney-client privilege, the physician-patient relationship involves **privileged communication.** This is information

Legal Brief WHEN THE PATIENT IS INCOMPETENT

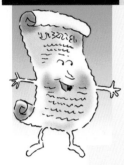

People who are mentally incompetent due to drug use, senility, or other mental disabilities can't enter into contracts. Because consent is a form of contract, this restriction also affects their ability to give consent for treatment. In these cases, the patient's legal guardian must provide consent. If the patient doesn't have a guardian, a court will appoint someone to act on the patient's behalf.

In general, **minors** (persons under 18 years of age) are also legally incompetent and consent must be obtained from the minor's parent or guardian. In some cases, however, minors are able to give consent.

- **Emancipated minors** are minors who are married, in the armed forces, or self-supporting. A court must determine whether a minor qualifies as self-supporting. The medical assistant should place a copy of this court order, marriage certificate, or proof of military status in the patient's medical record.

- **Mature minors** are minors judged competent enough to understand and make their own treatment decisions in certain circumstances. Usually, these circumstances involve treatment for birth control, pregnancy, drug or alcohol abuse, sexually transmitted diseases, or psychological evaluation. Laws regarding mature minors and consent vary from state to state.

Even when a minor can't legally give consent, the physician should still try to involve the patient in the caregiving process to the extent of the child's ability to understand.

that's protected by law from being disclosed except in very limited circumstances. In a medical setting, the doctrine of privileged communication applies *unless:*

- the patient **waives** (gives up) the protection or privilege
- the information is subpoenaed by court order (you read about this process in Chapter 2)
- the information is needed to carry out the patient's treatment and care, or to be paid for by the patient's health plan
- disclosure of the information is required by law

You'll read more about releasing patient information in Chapter 7.

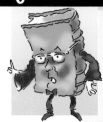

By the Book PROTECTING PATIENT PRIVACY

Here are some practices you can follow in your daily activities to help safeguard patients' privacy.

- Don't leave patients' medical records in areas where patients or other office visitors can see them.

- Use extreme caution when giving any information about a patient to someone who calls on the phone. It's often difficult or impossible to verify that the caller is authorized to have the information. It's better to err on the side of caution and avoid releasing the information until you've verified that it's okay to do so. Once you provide information, you can't take it back.

- When you're talking with a patient on the phone, use the patient's name as little as possible in case others might overhear you. Also, speak softly to keep others from overhearing the conversation. It's best if the employees who are responsible for answering the phone are not in an area where patients can overhear conversations. Thus, in some offices, an employee other than the receptionist will answer the phone.

- When you can't reach a patient on the phone, simply leave a message asking him to call the physician's office. Be sure to include the office phone number in your message. Don't reveal the reason for your call or even the physician's specialty or type of practice.

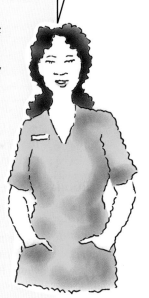

In Chapter 7, you'll learn about precautions to follow when releasing patient records.

LEGALLY REQUIRED DISCLOSURES

Besides her duties to her patients, a physician has responsibilities to the community. In certain circumstances, a physician must report specific patient information to legal authorities.

Vital Statistics

Vital statistics are data about the general population. They include records of births, deaths, marriages, and divorces. These records are used by the government to track population trends.

Physicians are required to report every baby they deliver. They do this by filing an official certificate of birth with the county in which the birth occurred. If the mother delivered in a hospital, the hospital will complete and file the birth certificate. But the physician must verify the information and sign it.

If a patient dies, the physician usually must complete and sign a death certificate reporting the date, time, place, and cause of death. The death certificate must also state how long the patient was under the physician's care and whether an **autopsy** was performed. (An autopsy is an examination of the body to determine the cause of death when a death is suspicious or the cause is unclear.)

In some cases, the law prohibits the physician from signing a patient's death certificate. These situations include the following:

- deaths at which the physician was not present or had not seen the patient within a certain length of time before the death

- deaths due to unknown causes

- violent deaths, including those from suicide and accidents

- deaths that are suspicious or possibly due to criminal actions

In these cases, a government official must complete the death certificate.

Public Health Reporting

Physicians must report patients who have communicable diseases that are considered a threat to the general population. A **communicable disease** is a disease that can be passed from one person to another. The list of reportable diseases varies from state to state. But all states require that the following diseases be reported to public health officials:

- tuberculosis, cholera, polio, meningitis, and rheumatic fever

- rubeola and rubella (types of measles)

- HIV and AIDS

- sexually transmitted diseases (STDs)

Reportable STDs vary from state to state, but they usually include the following:

- syphilis

- gonorrhea

- genital warts

- chlamydia

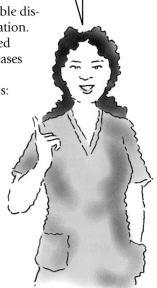

Although physicians are required to report certain STDs, a patient's diagnosis must be kept confidential. The public health department—not the physician's office—is responsible for notifying a patient's past or current sexual partners about possible infection.

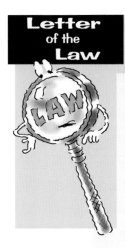

THE NATIONAL CHILDHOOD VACCINE INJURY ACT

The National Childhood Vaccine Injury Act requires that physicians report all adverse (harmful) reactions to any vaccinations they administer for the following diseases:

- measles, mumps, and rubella (MMR)
- diphtheria, pertussis, and tetanus (DPT)
- polio (both live and inactive vaccine)
- hepatitis B
- influenza type B
- varicella (chicken pox)

To make this reporting helpful, physicians are required to record the following information in the chart of each patient who receives one of these vaccines:

- the date the vaccine was given
- the vaccine manufacturer and lot number
- the name, address, and title of the person who gave the vaccine

Reporting Abuse and Neglect

All 50 states have laws that require physicians to notify authorities when they see injuries or other conditions in children and elderly patients that suggest the patients are being abused or neglected. Signs of these conditions include malnutrition or bruises, broken bones, and other injuries that can't be satisfactorily explained by the patient.

Child Abuse

In all states, suspected or validated child abuse must be reported by phone or in person at once, followed by a written report, usually within 72 hours. The law protects the physician from any criminal or civil liability for making the report.

Spousal Abuse

Most states do not require a physician to report spousal abuse unless the patient states that his injuries were the result of abuse. However, all states have laws to protect the victims of domestic violence.

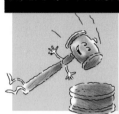

What's the Verdict?   DISCLOSING PATIENT INFORMATION

A patient applies to an insurance company for a life insurance policy. To determine the patient's state of health, the company requires a physician's examination before the policy can be issued. The physician discovers that the patient suffers from heart disease. The patient asks the physician not to report this finding to the insurance company. When the physician does so anyway, the patient sues him for violating the confidentiality of the patient's medical information.

The Verdict: The physician's action did not violate patient confidentiality. Because the examination was performed at the insurance company's request (and the insurance company was paying), the patient should have expected that the findings would be reported to the insurance company. By going ahead with the exam, the patient gave his implied consent to the release of the exam's results to the insurance company.

Elder Abuse

All states have systems for reporting the neglect and the physical, sexual, or financial abuse of older adults, whether at home or in institutions. Although reporting is voluntary in some states, most require physicians to report suspected elder abuse. However, some forms of emotional abuse and neglect are not crimes in all states.

Other Reportable Injuries

In all states, a physician must immediately report to the police any patient she's treated whose injuries appear to have resulted from an act of violence. In most states, the following conditions require reporting:

- gunshot wounds
- stab wounds
- rape or evidence that suggests rape
- other evidence that suggests the patient has been assaulted

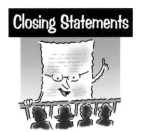
Closing Statements

- Patients have the right to a choice of providers, to respect and nondiscrimination, to participation in treatment decisions, and to the privacy of their medical information. They also have the responsibility to be honest with the physician and to cooperate with their care by following the physician's instructions.

- Physicians have the right to refuse to treat certain patients and the responsibility to provide the patients they do choose to treat with the proper standard of care.

- Managed-care organizations, such as HMOs and PPOs, have become common as health care plans try to control the costs of medical care. Some critics claim that managed care has adversely affected the rights and responsibilities of physicians and patients and has reduced the quality of care.

- A three-party contract between the physician, the patient, and the patient's health plan affects how the physician is paid for the services provided. Contracts between the physician and managed-care plans affect how services are delivered and what the physician may charge for those services.

- Consent is central to patient rights and to the physician-patient relationship. The patient's involvement in treatment decisions requires the patient's informed consent.

- Confidentiality is another important aspect of the physician-patient relationship. The privacy of medical information is needed to ensure the patient's full cooperation with the physician in diagnosing and caring for the patient's medical needs.

- Under some circumstances, the physician is obligated to report the patient's medical information to authorities. These situations include reporting births, deaths, and certain communicable diseases. They also involve reporting patient injuries that suggest violent crimes or possible child, spousal, or elder abuse.

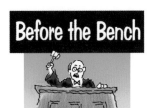
Before the Bench

Answer the following multiple-choice questions.

1. A patient's rights include all of the following *except:*
   a. right to privacy.
   b. right to refuse treatment.
   c. right to consent to treatment.
   d. right to a cure.

2. A patient's responsibilities for his care include:
   a. being honest in his communications with the physician.

    b. following the physician's instructions.

    c. paying for the services the physician provides.

    d. all of the above

3. Which right has been limited by the growth of managed care?

    a. physicians' right to refuse to treat a patient

    b. patients' right to choose their health care provider

    c. physicians' right to choose their medical specialty

    d. patients' right to the privacy of their health information

4. A physician who receives a set payment in advance to cover all the care she will provide to a patient is most likely participating in:

    a. an HMO.

    b. a PPO.

    c. a POS.

    d. an EPO.

5. The *main* purpose of managed care is to:

    a. provide a patient with a greater choice of physicians.

    b. improve the standard of care in the practice of medicine.

    c. control the costs of treating a patient.

    d. make it easier for a patient to see a specialist.

6. What type of consent is a patient giving by signing a consent-for-treatment form?

    a. expressed consent

    b. implied consent

    c. informed consent

    d. all of the above

7. Informed consent is *not* required for:

    a. minor surgery.

    b. experimental procedures.

    c. risky treatments.

    d. routine procedures.

8. In which situation is a parent's consent usually *not* needed to treat a minor patient?

    a. if the minor is incompetent

    b. if the minor is seeking birth control

    c. if the minor understands the risks of treatment

    d. if the minor agrees to the treatment

9. When is the privacy of a patient's information *not* protected?

    a. when the physician is required to report it by law

    b. when a member of the patient's family requests it

    c. when it's information that's unrelated to the patient's
       health
    d. all of the above

10. In most states, a physician must notify authorities if he
    treats a patient for:
    a. a gunshot wound.
    b. a sexually transmitted disease.
    c. injuries that suggest child or elder abuse.
    d. all of the above

Chapter 7

ALL ABOUT
MEDICAL RECORDS

Chapter Checklist

- Identify who owns a medical chart and who owns the information in the chart

- Explain why medical records are necessary

- Explain in general terms how electronic medical records are recorded

- Discuss the information required for every entry in the medical chart and why it is important

- Describe the procedure for making corrections in the medical chart

- Discuss what is required to release patient information

- Determine the minimum time medical records are to be kept

- Describe the proper procedure for disposal of medical records

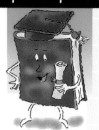

Chapter Competencies

- Establish and maintain the medical record (CAAHEP 3.c.2.c.)

- Document appropriately (CAAHEP 3.c.2.d.)

- Document accurately (ABHES 5.b.)

- Identify and respond to issues of confidentiality (CAAHEP 3.c.2.a.)

- Perform within legal and ethical boundaries (CAAHEP 3.c.2.b.)

- Maintain confidentiality at all times (ABHES 1.b.)

- Use appropriate guidelines when releasing records or information (ABHES 5.c.)

At their most basic level, patient records are the patient's history with the medical office. That's because they hold the record of every encounter the office has had with every patient. This wealth of information makes patient records a critical resource in the practice of medicine.

In many offices the medical assistant is **custodian** of the medical records—the person charged with their care. In this chapter, you'll learn how medical records are organized, what's in them, who has a right to that information, and under what conditions that information may be accessible. You'll also learn about charting in a medical record and when medical records should be retained or destroyed.

The Patient's Medical Record

A patient's **medical record** is the written record documenting all medical care the office has provided to the patient. It includes:

- the patient's personal information, including name, date of birth, Social Security number, and contact information— that is, the patient's address and phone number
- the patient's medical history; this information is of two types:
  1. *Subjective information* is information the patient provides, such as a complaint of a backache. This information is subject to the patient's descriptions and is difficult to prove.
  2. *Objective information* is information that can be measured, such as the patient's height, blood pressure, lab results, or vital signs.
- the patient's current diagnosis and treatment
- all correspondence related to the patient, including results of outside tests, letters sent and received, and a record of phone calls to and from the patient

A patient's medical record is sometimes called the patient's *chart.* Besides being the history of the patient's relationship with the office, it's also a legal document. In fact, it's the only official, legal record of what was done—and not done—to and for the patient. For this reason, it must be carefully handled and managed.

CAREFUL MANAGEMENT OF MEDICAL RECORDS

Here are some tips on careful handling and management of medical records.

- The information in the medical record must be thorough and accurate. The medical record is no place for noting your personal opinions of the patient or what you expect the patient's diagnosis to be. Document only the facts.
- Each patient's record must be properly filed so it can be easily retrieved when needed.
- All patients' medical records must be properly stored, even after patients stop seeing the physician, in case a patient's care ever becomes the subject of a legal dispute.

YOURS AND MINE

Who owns a patient's medical record? The answer is complicated. Whoever creates the record has the property right to it. (A **property right** is the right of ownership.) For instance, a hospital owns the medical records of its past and present patients. A physician's office owns the medical records of the patients the physician has seen. But the *information* in a medical record is the *patient's* property.

This ownership situation is the reason that, in most cases, a patient has a right to read and get a copy of his medical record. It's also why, with only a few exceptions, the patient's permission must be obtained before information in his record can be shared with others. (You'll read about the exceptions to these patient rights later in this chapter.)

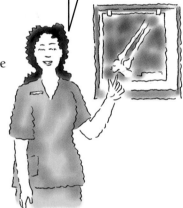

X-rays and other tests usually belong to the office, not to the patient. That's because they're considered part of the medical record.

A RECORD OF MANY USES

One purpose for medical records has already been hinted at: to provide evidence that can be used in a malpractice suit. A well-kept medical record is often a physician's best defense against an accusation that malpractice took place. Or the patient might try to use his medical record as evidence to show that malpractice actually did occur.

This is why it's so important that all interactions with patients be accurately and thoroughly documented in their

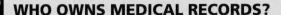

What's the Verdict? WHO OWNS MEDICAL RECORDS?

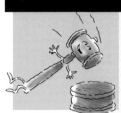

A physician is employed by a large clinic. When she resigns to start her own practice, she takes the medical records of the clinic patients she's been treating and places them in her new office. The clinic demands that she return the records. The physician argues that since she was the physician for the patients whose records she removed, their records are her property.

The Verdict: The physician must return the records to the clinic. Because she was an employee of the clinic, the records are not her property. Rather, the records are the property of the clinic—her employer at the time she was seeing the patients. Patients who want this particular physician to continue caring for them must sign a records release/transfer and have the clinic transfer their records to her new office.

charts. This includes all phone and in-person conversations with each patient, any cancelled or missed appointments, and, of course, all care and other services provided.

You've read elsewhere in this book about the old saying in health care that if it's not in the chart, it didn't happen. From a legal standpoint this is quite true! Juries tend to believe what happened if it's documented in the medical record at the time. On the other hand, juries tend *not* to believe something took place if it's not recorded in the patient's chart.

Other uses of the medical record and the information it contains include the following:

- allowing better management of the patient's care by providing information about the patient's past conditions, treatment, and the outcome of that treatment
- providing data that allow government officials and other researchers to compile statistics on birth rates, deaths, communicable diseases, and other matters of concern to the public health

IT'S NOT YOUR FATHER'S MEDICAL RECORD!

For decades, medical records have consisted of sheets of 8½-by-11-inch paper attached inside cardboard folders that look something like file folders. Notes on the patient's visit were recorded on blank forms inside the record. As the patient returned for more care, more blank forms were added as needed to document these return visits. Reports of test results, consultation reports from other physicians, and other materials from "outside" sources were added to the medical record as they arrived in the office.

Many medical offices continue to use these paper charts today. But more and more offices are now using **electronic medical records.** In this type of record system, patients' medical records are kept in an electronic file. Medical offices can purchase special computer software from medical software manufacturers to create these electronic records.

In an electronic medical record, notes about patients' visits and treatment are entered into their record using the computer screen and keyboard, PDAs, or other electronic devices rather than being written in a paper chart by hand. A scanner can be used to transfer reports, letters, and other paper documents into the patient's medical record on the computer.

However, test results and much other outside information already is often available by computer—through e-mail, attachments to e-mail, access to databases, and so on. In such cases, the scanning step would not be necessary to place information from other sources into the patient's electronic chart.

TECHNOLOGY AND THE FUTURE OF MEDICAL RECORDS

Advances in technology allow medical records systems to continue to evolve. For example, many people now carry "health cards" with magnetic strips that provide the following:

- the name and contact information for the person's physician
- the person's health insurance plan information
- the person's blood type and major medical conditions
- all medications the person is taking
- any allergies the person has
- a code that allows medical personnel access to a computer database, so the patient's full medical record is immediately available

The popularity of tiny portable computer hard drives called flash drives also allows a patient to carry her entire medical record on her key chain or in her purse or pocket. She simply has to have the physician's office copy her electronic medical record from the office computer to her flash drive.

In 2004 the U.S. Food and Drug Administration (FDA) approved the use of a chip that can be scanned with a handheld scanner. The size of the tip of a ballpoint pen, the chip can be implanted in a person's arm in a quick, simple office surgery under local anesthesia. When scanned, the chip gives any physician access to that patient's record on a computer database.

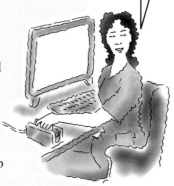

New technology allows medical professionals to access detailed patient information with the swipe of a card.

It's not hard to imagine a time when technology will exist to allow a patient to have all her health information on a chip in a medical bracelet or under her skin. A scanner in the physician's office would pull up the patient's medical record on the computer when she arrives for her appointment. The scanner would also transfer the updated medical record from the computer to the patient's chip at the end of every visit!

On the (Medical) Record

The contents of a patient's medical record will depend somewhat on the medical office's specialty. For example, medical records in a dermatology practice are likely to contain photographs. Many dermatologists document treatment with before and after photos of patients' skin.

But regardless of the service provided, most medical records will contain the following items:

- the patient's identifying and contact information that you read about earlier in this chapter, as well as the patient's e-mail address, place of employment, and work phone number, if appropriate
- the patient's insurance information, including the name of the health plan, the policy holder and his relationship to the patient, the policy and group numbers, and a photocopy of the front and back of the patient's insurance card
- a photocopy of the patient's driver's license
- the patient's emergency contact information, including name, address, and necessary phone numbers; similar

information should be recorded for the patient's legal representative in case the patient is not able to give consent for treatment

- the name and billing address of the person responsible for paying the bill
- the patient's health history
- the dates and times of each appointment, including the patient's symptoms and reason for making it
- the examination performed by the physician at each appointment, as well as the physician's assessment, diagnosis, and notes on the patient's progress
- the treatment provided at each appointment, as well as notes on instructions to the patient and on prescriptions written for new medications or refills
- x-ray reports, lab reports, and all other test results, including the strips from any ECGs
- reports from any other physicians consulted on a specific case
- all consent forms signed for treatments or procedures
- notes on all phone calls to and from the patient, including the date, reason for the call, and what took place; unsuccessful attempts to call the patient should also be noted, including their outcome—such as "no answer" or any messages left
- a record of all copies made of the medical record, including the date, what was sent, and to whom it was sent
- notes on the patient's condition when treatment is stopped, including the reason for terminating treatment

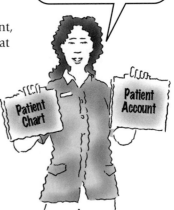

Billing records are not part of the medical record. They're kept in a separate patient financial account.

Patient Chart

Patient Account

KEEPING IT CREDIBLE

A credible medical record means that the information it contains is correct. This is especially important because, if a legal dispute over care arises, the medical record may be introduced as evidence in court. A well-kept medical record is likely to be more convincing to a jury than the testimony of witnesses trying to remember something that may have happened long ago. Remember that legible handwriting is an important part of a well-kept chart. There have been instances in court where the physician himself is not able to decipher what he has written in a patient's chart.

The medical record can even help prevent a lawsuit from happening in the first place. Suppose a patient goes to a lawyer about the care he's received. The first thing the lawyer will do is get a copy of the patient's medical record. She'll then hire an expert—usually a physician or a nurse—to go over the record, looking for evidence of malpractice. A credible medical record may satisfy the reviewer that the patient has no case.

On the other hand, a poorly kept medical record, with incomplete or missing information, can make a lawsuit more likely. For example, suppose the physician's notes in the chart show that blood tests were ordered. But no test results are in the record. That's likely to arouse suspicions that:

- the tests were not done
- the test results were overlooked when treating the patient
- the test results were removed from the record to cover up an error

Any of these possibilities would strengthen a case that malpractice might have occurred.

KEEPING IT CURRENT

One of the keys to maintaining a credible medical record is keeping it current. This means placing information received from outside sources into the patient's medical record soon after it arrives. Depending on your office's medical record system, that can involve these tasks:

- filing paper reports in a paper chart
- scanning paper reports into an electronic medical record
- moving reports received by computer into the proper patient's electronic record
- printing reports received by computer and filing the paper printouts in the patient's paper chart

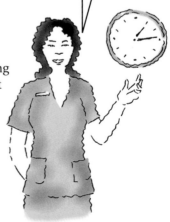

When it comes to charting, time is of the essence! Document events in a patient's chart as soon as possible to ensure completeness and accuracy.

Another important part of keeping a record current is timely **documentation** or "**charting**." You should enter your notes in a patient's medical record as soon as possible after the event you're documenting. Prompt charting means that you don't have to rely on your memory of something that took place hours or days ago. That helps make the note more complete and accurate.

Timely charting also helps make sure that events are recorded in the order in which they happened. Suppose, for example, you wait several hours to write something in a patient's medical record. You then discover that the nurse has already documented something that happened with that patient later in the day. Now your chart note will be out of chronological order. If there's ever a problem, this may make the chart less credible. It may look like your note was added later as an attempt to cover something up.

TELLING THE WHOLE STORY

When making notes in a patient's chart, be sure to document the details of the event. For example, don't just write, *Patient phoned office.* Include a summary of what the patient said and your response to the patient. Use the patient's own words, in quotation marks, whenever possible.

Although you want to be sure to include all of the important facts in your documentation, you also want to be concise. Being concise means giving a lot of information in as few words as possible. Documentation should be brief as well as complete.

Finally, your writing should be readable and the note easy to understand. Words that are not legible or are poorly chosen can change a note's meaning, depending on how they're read. For example, the words *hyperglycemia* and *hypoglycemia* look similar, but mean different things. Failing to clearly write the intended word can make a big difference!

OOPS, I MADE A MISTAKE!

Nobody's perfect. There'll be times when you make a mistake when charting in a patient's medical record. Most electronic medical record programs have safeguards that help you make corrections in the proper way. But if you're using a paper system, here's what to do when correcting a mistake in the chart.

1. Draw a single line through the error. Make sure that the error remains readable.

2. Enter the correct information above or below the line or in the margin next to the note. If you need more space to make the correction, attach another sheet of paper with the correction on it. Then note at the site of the mistake, "See attachment A" to indicate where the correction can be found.

3. Enter the date, time, and your initials next to the correction.

It's also a good idea to ask the physician or another staff member to witness the correction by initialing it as well.

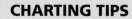

By the Book **CHARTING TIPS**

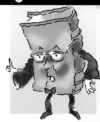

Here are some other guidelines to follow when making entries in a patient's medical record. Most of them apply to electronic medical records as well as to paper charts.

- Make sure you have the correct patient's medical record before beginning your note.

- The patient's name should appear on each page of the record, whether it's a paper page or a "page" in an electronic record.

- You must record the time and date for each entry you make and place your initials at the end of your note. This prevents someone from adding to your note later.

- Never initial a note that someone else has written, either with your own initials or those of the note writer. It's unethical to sign a medical record for someone else, and it can also be illegal to do so.

- Make sure that all medical terms you use are correctly spelled. Many terms have similar spellings, and an incorrect spelling could change the meaning of your note. If you're not sure, use your medical dictionary to confirm the spelling of a difficult term.

- Use only medical abbreviations that are generally known or that are common to your office. Your office should maintain a list of acceptable abbreviations and their meanings.

- Document all phone calls to and from the patient and all missed appointments.

- When charting in paper records, use only a black pen. Black ink shows up best when records are photocopied.

- Never state opinions or judgments, use sarcasm or humor, or make personal remarks about the patient in your notes.

> It's especially important to not make up your own shorthand or abbreviations for use in medical records. Use only those abbreviations recognized by your office.

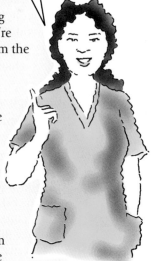

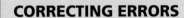

Legal Brief | CORRECTING ERRORS

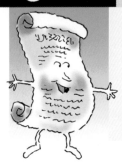

Never erase, white out, or otherwise completely block out a charting error. It's important that all errors in a medical record can be easily read. If they can't, it might look like someone has deliberately tried to get rid of damaging information. This suspicion could hurt the physician's case if the record ever becomes evidence in a malpractice suit.

Ideally, charting errors should be corrected when they're made. If an error isn't discovered until later, it should be corrected at that time. However, problems can arise if a long time passes between the original entry and the date of the correction. In the event of a lawsuit, such corrections can make a chart less credible by creating suspicion of a cover-up or fraud.

MEDICAL RECORDS FRAUD

The threat of a lawsuit for malpractice, abandonment, or some other health care–related issue might tempt some health care providers to alter the patient's chart after the fact. Health care providers may be tempted to:

- change information in the chart to weaken the patient's case
- add new, false information to the record to strengthen the provider's defense
- remove documents from the chart that might weaken the provider's case

Altering a medical record in these ways is *always* a bad idea, and not only that, it's illegal! Health care providers who attempt medical fraud rarely get away with it. That's because everyone in the office must go along with it, making them accessories to the fraud. It's almost certain that some employees won't want to take that risk, and that their personal and professional ethics will cause them to stand up and expose the fraud.

Once it's known that the record has been altered, the defendant's case is destroyed. That's because the defendant's action suggests that he's guilty of something.

When medical records fraud is discovered, most malpractice insurance companies will automatically try to **settle** the case. That is, the company will try to get the patient to accept money to drop the suit. If the case does go to court, the jury is likely to award greater damages to the patient because of the fraud.

My Record and My Rights

You've read about the confidentiality of patients' health information in Chapter 6 and in several earlier chapters. The protection of a patient's privacy is one of the most important legal and ethical responsibilities entrusted to health care workers. The legal and ethical responsibilities extend to the patient's medical record, too.

LET ME HAVE IT!

In general, patients have a right to review their medical records and request that necessary corrections be made. They also have a right to get copies of their medical records, although the physician's office usually can charge a fee to cover the copying costs. Many offices will provide the first copy for free as a service to the patient. A few states have laws requiring that medical offices provide patients with one free copy before they can charge for additional copies. When a patient is reviewing her medical record, a member of the medical office staff should be present the entire time. Never leave a patient alone with her chart. If the patient is contemplating suing the physician and you've left the chart with the patient, she may have an opportunity to alter her medical records to strengthen her case.

Limits on a Patient's Rights

Whether the patient's copy is free or not, the office can set a reasonable time limit for providing it. A patient has no right to require that a copy of her record be provided immediately upon making her request.

Also, the physician may not allow a patient to have her record if he thinks that seeing something in it might cause the patient harm. This concern usually applies to patients who have mental or emotional problems. The legal principle that lets a physician use his professional judgment to deny this right is called the **doctrine of professional discretion.** It's why you should never let a patient see her record without getting the physician's permission first.

When the Patient Is a Minor

In general, the legal principles that apply to minors and consent for treatment (which you read about in Chapter 6) also apply to medical records.

- Small children have no right to their records. However, a parent or guardian has the same rights as if she were the patient. That is, the parent or guardian has a right to know the information in the child's chart and to decide who else should have it.

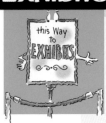

Exhibits

TECHNOLOGY AND CONFIDENTIALITY

Medical offices rely on various kinds of technology to store, maintain, and share patients' medical records. Here are some guidelines to follow when using these devices to help protect the confidentiality of patients' records.

- *Electronic files.* The computer files that contain patients' medical records should be password protected so that unauthorized persons can't gain access to them. Each employee authorized to work with medical records should have a unique login name and password. Computers should track and store a record of who logs into the files, when they did so, and for how long.

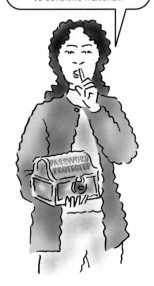

Never share your login or password with coworkers. Each staff member should have his own login name to gain access to sensitive material.

- *Computers.* Position computer monitors so that others can't see what's on the screen. Also, never leave a patient's record open on the screen. Close the record when you're finished with it, or if you have to leave the computer for some reason.

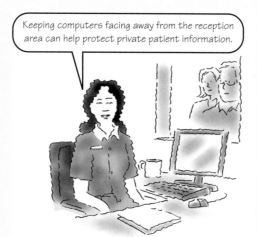

Keeping computers facing away from the reception area can help protect private patient information.

- *Printers.* Do not send electronic medical records to a printer in an area where unauthorized persons might see the printouts. Also, never leave a printer unattended when printing patient records. If you print pages you decide you don't need, shred them. Don't ever just discard them in the trash.

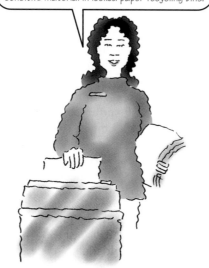

If your office doesn't have a shredder, talk to the office manager about how you should dispose of sensitive material. Some medical offices use outside shredding companies; in this case, place sensitive material in locked paper-recycling bins.

- *Copiers.* When photocopying medical records, don't leave the originals or copies unattended in the copier where others might see them. Any copies that are not needed after copying should be shredded. This also applies to copies or partial copies removed from the copier if it jams.

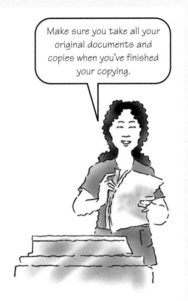

Make sure you take all your original documents and copies when you've finished your copying.

If you receive a phone call that another medical office is faxing over a patient's medical records, wait by the fax machine until this sensitive material safely arrives. Then file the paperwork as necessary.

- *Fax machines.* When sending a fax, first call the receiver to verify that you have the correct fax number before faxing medical records. This also alerts the receiver that confidential materials are on the way. This alert is especially important if the receiver's fax machine is in an area where unauthorized persons might see the fax. Also, don't leave the original records unattended in your fax machine while they are being transmitted. Finally, use a cover sheet that includes your name and phone number and reads: "Confidential material to addressee only. Please notify sender if this fax is received in error."

- Mature minors have control over those parts of their medical record that include treatment for which they can give legal consent. Parents can't be given any such information from the patient's record without the mature minor's consent.

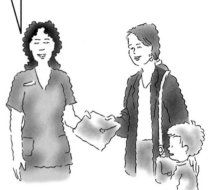

When a child's parents are divorced, the parent who has custody is the one who should authorize release of the child's medical records.

- Emancipated minors have the same rights to their records as adult patients do. This includes the right to decide who else can have the information in them. The parent of an emancipated minor can't have a copy of the medical record without the minor's permission.

RELEASING INFORMATION

With a few exceptions, a patient's medical record may not be **disclosed** (made known) without the patient's consent. This restriction applies to family members, friends, and employers—as well

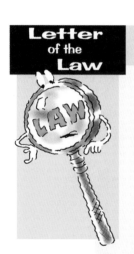

Letter of the Law

42 CFR PART 2

An administrative law issued by the U.S. Department of Health and Human Services (HHS) prohibits the disclosure of any records that reveal a patient is being treated for drug or alcohol abuse. The rule is the Confidentiality of Alcohol and Drug Abuse Patient Records Regulation, but it's better known as "42 CFR Part 2," which stands for its location in the federal administrative law code.

The following are the *only* exceptions to this rule:

- when the patient signs a release allowing the disclosure
- when suspected child abuse is involved
- when the patient commits a crime against treatment center workers or property
- when the information is needed to aid patient's treatment in a medical emergency

Persons who violate 42 CFR Part 2 are subject to fines under criminal law.

as to others who may have a legitimate interest in the patient's health.

If a patient wants someone to know what's in his medical record, he must sign a form that gives the physician permission to disclose the information. The form must indicate which information he's consenting to release and to whom. Unless the form states otherwise, the disclosure has no time limit.

A copy of the signed form should be given to the patient and another copy should be placed in the patient's chart. A patient can always withdraw his consent to release his records. If he does this, the information can no longer be disclosed.

WHEN CONSENT IS NOT NEEDED

There are times when the information in a patient's medical record can be disclosed without the patient's consent. You've already read about some of these exceptions in earlier chapters, such as:

- when a court issues a subpoena for a medical record (Chapter 2)

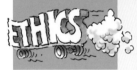

Ethics in Action   **KEEPING RECORDS CONFIDENTIAL**

Professional ethics require you to respect the confidentiality of patients' medical information. Follow these practices in handling patient's charts and the information in them.

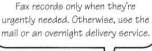

Fax records only when they're urgently needed. Otherwise, use the mail or an overnight delivery service.

- Don't leave paper charts in areas where unauthorized people could read them. This also applies to reports and other items that are awaiting filing in patients' charts.

- Don't discuss any information in a patient's record—even with authorized people—in places where unauthorized people might overhear the conversation. And never give any information from a patient's record to someone who's not authorized to have it.

- When fulfilling authorized requests for information from a medical record, be sure to provide no more than what's asked for. Apply this safeguard to the records you copy or fax, as well as to any information you give out over the phone.

- when the patient's health plan needs information to make a decision on paying for the patient's care (Chapter 3)
- when another health care provider needs the records to treat or test the patient, or to consult about the patient with the patient's physician (Chapter 3)
- when public health and safety laws require the physician to report the information to authorities (Chapter 6)

There are several other situations where the patient's consent is not required.

The Military Exception

If a person is on active duty in the armed forces, no consent to release his records is needed if the military makes an official request for them. This exception also applies to his records of treatment when he was a civilian. However, it does not apply to the records of the dependents of military personnel.

Exceptions for Investigations

Authorities who enforce federal and state laws that regulate health care do not need patients' permission to review their medical records. For example, government investigators may want to determine whether the office is complying with drug, Medicare, or Medicaid laws. They must be allowed to see any patient records they request during their investigation.

Can Law Enforcement Officers Access Records?

Can law enforcement officers, such as the local police or the FBI, have access to a patient's medical records? Generally, the answer is "no." This is not an answer that officers usually want to hear, especially if they're investigating the patient for a crime. Always check with the physician first. But unless she tells you to do otherwise, hold your ground.

It's best to require that officers get a warrant to see the records, rather than surrender them voluntarily. A **warrant** is a written order from a judge that gives police the authority to do something. That protects you, and the physician, from being sued by the patient for violating medical confidentiality.

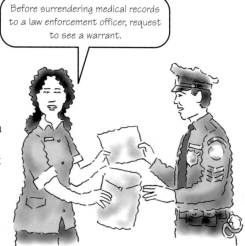

Before surrendering medical records to a law enforcement officer, request to see a warrant.

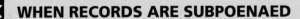

By the Book WHEN RECORDS ARE SUBPOENAED

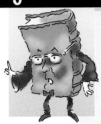

If a physician is sued for malpractice, a medical assistant may become responsible for complying with the *subpoena duces tecum*. This is a court order requiring certain records to be brought to court to be used as evidence in a trial. Follow these guidelines when complying with a *subpoena duces tecum*.

- Check the subpoena to make sure the **docket number** of the case and the name of the court are on it. (The docket number is a number that identifies the case in court records.)
- Check office records to verify that the plaintiff named on the subpoena is or was a patient of the physician.
- Call the court to verify the trial date and time that are listed on the subpoena.
- Notify the physician that a subpoena has been received. (Subpoenas may be served by a law enforcement officer, a hired process server, or by certified mail.) Then, notify the physician's malpractice insurance company or her attorney if she tells you to do so.
- Gather the subpoenaed records. Make sure you have everything that's been subpoenaed. Also, check to make sure that you're providing only what's been subpoenaed and nothing more. Keep these records in a secure area.
- Check all the subpoenaed records to make sure they're complete. But never alter any of them in any way. Make a record of the number of pages being provided.
- Provide only photocopies of the subpoenaed records, if possible. If the subpoena requires original records, make photocopies to keep in the office.
- Be prepared to provide sworn testimony about preparing the records, if the court requires it.

After She's Gone . . .

Of course, a current patient's medical records should all be kept as long as the office continues treating the patient. But what should you do about the records of former patients?

Some states have laws that require how long medical records must be retained. If your state doesn't, medical records should be kept at least until the statute of limitations on filing a malpractice suit has expired.

RECORDS RETENTION

As you read in Chapter 2, state statutes of limitations are often only two or three years. It's not unusual for some patients to wait that long between visits to the physician. For this reason, most physicians keep an adult patient's medical record for ten years from the date of the last entry in it. In some states, the physician will keep a minor's records for two years after the patient (or former patient) becomes an adult.

Some physicians choose to keep medical records forever. That's because of statutes of limitations that let minor patients bring suit after they become adults—or statutes that don't start to run until the evidence of possible malpractice is first discovered.

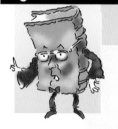

By the Book AMERICAN HEALTH INFORMATION MANAGEMENT ASSOCIATION GUIDELINES

The American Health Information Management Association (AHIMA) is a professional organization that's dedicated to improving health care by advancing the best practices and standards for health information management. With this goal in mind, the AHIMA offers the following guidelines for retaining medical records:

- adult patient records— ten years after the last encounter

- minors' patient records— the state age of maturity plus the state statute of limitations

- diagnostic images (such as photographs and x-rays)—five years

- birth and death registration records— permanently

These recommendations apply to electronic medical records as well as to paper charts.

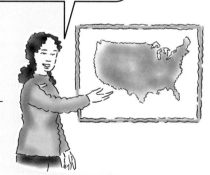

Let your state law be your guide on retaining patient records—or follow AHIMA guidelines.

STORAGE AND DESTRUCTION

The paper records of former patients can be stored in the office, separate from the files of current records. But, over time, the space required for records storage will grow. Many physicians rent storage space off-site. Be sure that any off-site storage space is climate controlled. Exposure to extreme heat, humidity, or damp conditions can damage records over time. Any exposure to water is likely to make paper records unreadable.

Some physicians have their old medical records photographed and stored on microfiche or microfilm. These images can also be stored on CD-ROMs or DVDs. Electronic records can be stored on CD-ROMs or DVDs, too.

Another choice for electronic storage is an external hard drive. These are separate, stand-alone hard drives that can be connected to the office computer. Once connected, the unused files can be transferred to the computer. The hard drive can then be disconnected and stored elsewhere.

The storage space required by any of these systems is quite small. This can allow the practice to store all its inactive records right in the medical office, where they're easily retrievable.

Records that have passed their retention deadlines can be destroyed. This should be done in a manner that makes them unreadable by any unauthorized person. The AHIMA offers guidelines in this area of record management, too.

- Paper records should be burned, shredded, or pulped beyond recognition.
- CD-ROMs, DVDs, microfilm, and microfiche should be pulverized.
- Hard drives should be overwritten.

Overwriting is an electronic process that wipes a hard drive clean. Simply deleting files from a hard drive allows the files to be recovered with special software programs. But overwriting makes it impossible to recover the information that was on the drive.

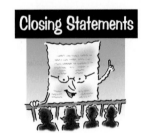

Closing Statements

- A medical record contains all the information a health care provider has gathered about a patient. A medical record belongs to the health care provider who created it, but the information it contains is the patient's property.
- Medical records allow better care by providing information about a patient's health history. By documenting treatment and other contact with a patient, the medical record can be a physician's best defense in a lawsuit. Medical records are also a valuable source of public health data.

- In the past, medical records have been paper records. Today, most medical offices create electronic medical records on a computer.

- A medical record should include the patient's personal and insurance information, health and treatment history, test results, consultation reports, appointment history, consent forms, and all communications with the patient. Properly kept medical records provide a good defense in legal disputes. Charts should be kept current, and all notes should be in chronological order. Documentation should reflect the patient's own words when possible, and the writing should be concise and clear. Each chart note should begin with the date and time and end with the writer's name or initials and credentials.

- You should correct charting mistakes by drawing a single line through the incorrect information and providing the correct information, the date and time of the correction, and your initials nearby. False corrections, adding false new information, and removing records from a chart are all crimes.

- In most cases, patients have a right to their medical records. With a few exceptions, a patient's records can't be released to others without the patient's permission. The patient must sign a form stating which records are authorized for release and to whom.

- Medical records of former patients should be kept at least until the statute of limitations on malpractice has expired. Some state laws may require that they be kept longer. Most physicians keep the medical records of adult patients for at least ten years.

- The proper method for disposing of records depends on the form in which they are stored. All records should be destroyed in a way that makes them unreadable.

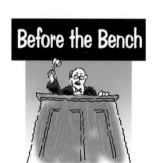

Before the Bench

Answer the following multiple-choice questions.

1. A medical record is legally owned by the:
   a. patient.
   b. physician.
   c. practice.
   d. state.

2. A patient's medical record:
   a. is a legal document.
   b. contains information that is confidential.
   c. can provide data for public health statistics.
   d. all of the above

3. A medical record contains all of the following *except:*
   a. the patient's past medical problems.
   b. the patient's payment record.
   c. the patient's insurance information.
   d. documentation of the patient's informed consent.

4. Entries in medical records should be made:
   a. as soon as possible after the patient leaves the office.
   b. at the end of each day.
   c. as soon as possible after the event being documented.
   d. when the physician tells you to do so.

5. Every entry in a medical record should be:
   a. accurate and complete.
   b. in chronological order.
   c. understandable to those who read it.
   d. all of the above

6. Which is a proper method for correcting errors in a medical record?
   a. thoroughly erase the incorrect information
   b. draw a single line through the incorrect information
   c. block out the incorrect information to make it unreadable
   d. all of the above

7. When must the office *always* obtain the patient's permission to release the information in her medical record?
   a. when the patient's employer asks about her condition
   b. when local police are investigating the patient for a crime
   c. when the patient is being treated for an STD
   d. when the patient's health insurance plan requests it

8. What is the minimum length of time an adult patient's record should be kept?
   a. until the patient is discharged
   b. until the statute of limitations has expired
   c. ten years
   d. forever

9. What is the *most* important factor to consider when storing medical records?
   a. the protection and security of the records
   b. the amount of storage space available
   c. the form in which the records will be stored
   d. the cost of storing the records

10. What is the proper way to destroy a medical record?
    a. shredding
    b. burning
    c. pulverizing or pulping
    d. all of the above

Chapter 8

WORKPLACE LAW

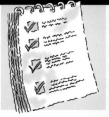

Chapter Checklist

- Discuss what "employment at will" means

- Name four laws that protect employees from discrimination

- List three questions an employer should not ask potential employees

- Define what the Federal Unemployment Tax Act (FUTA) is, how it affects the employee, and who pays

- Identify what constitutes sexual harassment

- Describe how OSHA applies to the medical office

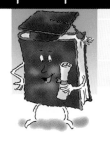

Chapter Competencies

- Perform within legal and ethical boundaries (CAAHEP 3.c.2.b.)

- Demonstrate knowledge of federal and state health care legislation and regulations (CAAHEP 3.c.2.f.)

- Evidence a responsible attitude (ABHES 1.g.)

Many federal and state laws apply to the workplace. They cover areas such as hiring and terminating employees, employee safety and welfare, pay and benefits, and other terms of employment. Federal laws usually apply only to businesses with a minimum number of workers—or to employees who work a certain number of hours per week, or a minimum number of weeks per year. State laws may fill these gaps in the federal protection of workers. They also may set requirements in some areas that are stricter than federal law.

In this chapter you'll learn about laws that affect the medical workplace. Since state laws vary from state to state, most of the laws you'll read about will be federal laws. It's important to know about these laws because they provide an environment for workers that's safe, humane, and fair.

You're Hired! . . . You're Fired!

In general, the common-law doctrine of employment at will governs the employer–employee relationship in most states. **Employment at will** means that either the employer or the employee can end the employment at any time and for any reason.

There are a few exceptions to the employment at will principle:

- Employees can't be fired for a reason prohibited by law— for example, because of their race or age. A person can't be refused employment for such illegal reasons, either.

- Employees who have employment contracts can't be fired, unless they breach the contract by violating its terms. The contract can be between the employer and the employee or the employer and a labor union to which the employee belongs.

GETTING HIRED

Employers must pay close attention to the law when hiring employees, as well as when firing them. Employers may gather information on a candidate's employment experience, education, and other things that are related to her ability to do the job.

An employer may also run a criminal background check and get a credit report on the candidate before hiring her. Both are common and acceptable hiring practices, especially if the job involves handling money or drugs. However, an employer's legal right to other personal information about a job seeker is much more limited.

Here are some of the things it's generally illegal to ask about, either on an employment application or in an interview.

- *Race, color, or national heritage.* As you've read, it's illegal to screen people on the basis of race.

- *Religion.* It's only legal to ask if the applicant's religious practices would interfere with work on any of the office's

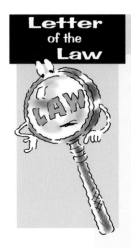

Letter of the Law

PREVENTING DISCRIMINATION

Discrimination is treating someone differently (and usually worse) than others because of some personal characteristic or practice. Both state and federal laws make discrimination in employment illegal. Here are some important antidiscrimination laws that apply to hiring and firing workers. Most of them apply to current workers as well, as you'll learn later in this chapter.

- *The Civil Rights Act of 1964.* Title VII of this law bans discrimination in hiring or firing on the basis of race, color, national origin, religion, or gender.

- *The Age Discrimination in Employment Act.* This 1967 law bans discrimination in hiring or firing on the basis of age. It protects persons age 40 and over and applies to employers with 20 or more employees.

- *The Pregnancy Discrimination Act.* This 1978 law makes it illegal to fire an employee because she's pregnant or has given birth, or because of a medical condition that's related to pregnancy and childbirth.

- *The Americans with Disabilities Act.* This 1990 law bans discrimination in hiring or firing because of a person's disability, as long as the abilities the person *does* have enable her to do the job.

Some states also have laws banning discrimination on the basis of a person's marital or parental status, mental limitations, physical appearance, or sexual orientation.

The Equal Employment Opportunity Commission (EEOC) is the federal government agency that investigates claims of employment discrimination. Someone who feels he's been discriminated against must contact the EEOC and let the agency try to settle the situation before he can sue the employer in court.

regular work days—for example, if the office is open on Saturdays or Sundays.

- *Gender.* It's illegal to ask, unless gender is critical to the duties of the job. For example, it would be legal to ask about an applicant's gender if the job were handing out towels in a women's locker room.

- *Date of birth or age.* It's only legal to ask if the applicant is under age 18. If the answer is *yes,* it's then legal to ask for his date of birth.

- *Birthplace.* It's illegal to ask where the applicant or any of her family members were born. That's because this information can be a clue to the applicant's national heritage. However, it *is* legal to ask if the applicant is a U.S. citizen.

- *Height and weight.* This information can only be gathered if it's important to performing the duties of the job.

- *Disabilities.* It's illegal to ask an applicant about any disabilities or diseases she may have. However, it *is* legal to ask if she has any physical limitations that would affect her ability to do the job.

- *Arrest record.* This is illegal to ask because it doesn't prove guilt. However, it *is* legal to ask if she's ever been convicted of a crime and the circumstances under which the crime happened.

- *Family status.* An applicant can't be asked if she is married, has children, is currently pregnant, or plans to have children.

Viewing and Interviewing

Of course, many of the items it's illegal to ask about on an application will become clear if the employer decides to inter-

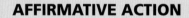

Legal Brief   AFFIRMATIVE ACTION

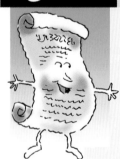

Affirmative action is a policy that gives preferred treatment to people from groups that have been discriminated against in the past. These disadvantaged groups include people with disabilities and certain minority groups. Women are a disadvantaged group in jobs where men have historically been hired.

At one time, employers were allowed, or even required, to reserve a certain number of positions for applicants from disadvantaged groups. However, the courts have ruled that this practice is illegal.

Today, employers are allowed to encourage members of disadvantaged groups to apply. They're also allowed to hire those applicants even if other applicants are better qualified. This type of affirmative action is not considered discrimination under the law.

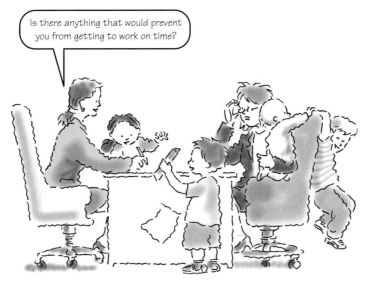

Is there anything that would prevent you from getting to work on time?

Poor attendance and tardiness are the top reasons medical assistants are fired.

view the applicant. For example, seeing the applicant in person will reveal gender, race, approximate age, and physical characteristics. A wedding ring would be a clue that the applicant is married. And she may mention her children during the course of the interview. But it's illegal to ask the applicant about any of these things if she doesn't volunteer the information herself.

It may seem harmless to mention that you have young children, or that you're currently going through a divorce, but think about it from the employer's standpoint. Imagine you're an employer, and you have to choose between two equally qualified applicants. One applicant has young children—children that might get sick, or be sent home from school on snow days, requiring the employee to leave work to care for them. The other applicant has college-aged children that will not require as much of the applicant's time. Many employers would make the easy choice and go with applicants who do not have as many outside-of-work demands on their time. By not volunteering information about your home and family, you do not give employers a reason to scratch you off their "potential hire" lists.

If an employer asks you an illegal question, you don't have to answer it. But be polite in your refusal. Don't say, "That's an illegal question, and I don't have to answer it!" A better response might be, "May I ask what that question has to do with the duties of the position?" Be aware, however, that even politely not answering such a question might cost you the job. Also, the fact that the employer asked an illegal question is not grounds to sue if you're not hired.

Pre-employment Screening

In addition to running a criminal records check and a credit check, an employer has the right to require a physical examination (at the employer's expense) before hiring you. To maintain patient confidentiality, the employer is allowed only to see the results of the physical exam, not your entire chart if the exam is done at the physician of your choosing. Most employers have contracted with an independent physician/ group to conduct all of their physical exams. Testing for drug use is also within an employer's legal rights, especially if you'll be working around drugs or using equipment that might cause injury to patients.

Many clinical sites, especially those accredited by the Joint Commission, require fingerprinting clearance cards. Fingerprinting is necessary to authenticate the identity and criminal history of health care professionals. The use of fingerprinting clearance cards (as part of a thorough background check) protects patients who can't defend or protect themselves against harmful or otherwise unsuitable treatment.

Many employers also require psychological and other tests as part of the hiring process. Such tests are allowed as long as they are measuring skills or abilities needed on the job. For example, an employer could test your skills as a medical assistant by asking you to complete a medical terminology test, data entry test, or instrument test prior to making a job offer. The employer may also require you to take a personality inventory to measure your ability to follow instructions and work well with others.

GETTING FIRED

You usually can't sue your employer simply because you were fired. You must have a **cause of action**—a legal basis for a lawsuit. For example, as you've just read, your employer can't fire you for a reason that's illegal, such as your race or your age. That would be discrimination, and discrimination is a cause of action.

In addition, even under employment at will, an employer can't fire you for no reason at all. The employer must have just cause to fire you. Being terminated without just cause is another cause of action for fired employees.

Just Cause, Not Just Because

Just cause is a legal reason for taking an action. For example, you may have done something that you shouldn't have done. Or you may *not* have done something that you should have done.

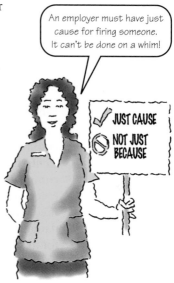

An employer must have just cause for firing someone. It can't be done on a whim!

A person can also sometimes be fired legally for reasons that aren't his fault. For example, suppose a physician leaves a group practice and its number of patients declines. The practice no longer needs as many medical assistants. That would give the employer just cause to let someone go.

Whatever the reason, an employer must show just cause if the employee challenges the firing decision. This means that the employer must be able to show just cause for its action. For the examples you've just read, documentation might be records showing that you were warned about your behavior or showing the drop in the number of patient appointments.

Wrongful Discharge

If your employer can't show a good reason for firing you, you may have grounds to sue the employer for wrongful discharge. **Wrongful discharge** is the tort of firing someone without just cause.

In addition to discrimination, there are a number of other reasons for which it's illegal to fire an employee. If an employee is released from employment for any of the following reasons, the employee may have been wrongfully "let go":

- for reporting illegal practices, such as billing fraud or safety violations; federal laws protect whistle-blowers from being punished by their employers, including punishment by firing.

- to prevent the employee from being eligible to collect pension or retirement benefits; doing this is a form of age discrimination.

- for joining a labor union or taking part in political activity; this includes trying to get coworkers to join a union. However, an employer *can* fire you if you do any of these things during the time when you should be working. Also, you may not wear campaign buttons and similar items on your work clothes.

- for refusing to take a drug test or a lie detector test; there are some exceptions to this protection, however.

- for exercising your right to freedom of speech; again, there are exceptions. For example, you can't be rude to patients or violate their confidentiality and expect to stay employed! Wearing pictures or other messages on your clothing that patients, coworkers, or your employer find offensive can also get you disciplined or even fired.

WRONGFUL DISCHARGE LAWSUITS

The Civil Rights Act of 1991 stiffened the penalties for employers who are sued for wrongful discharge. The Civil Rights Act of 1964 allowed plaintiffs to receive only compensatory damages for the loss of income and the emotional pain they had suffered by having been illegally fired. The 1991 act makes it possible to obtain punitive damages from the employer—to punish the employer for its behavior and discourage other employers from behaving that way, too.

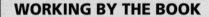

Legal Brief   WORKING BY THE BOOK

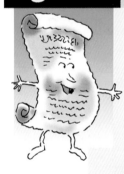

Many employers provide employees with a handbook that lists the employer's work practices and policies. Employee handbooks generally cover topics such as:

- work hours and paid holidays
- vacation, sick, and personal time and its use
- proper dress in the workplace
- guidelines for correct behavior
- procedures for handling improper employee behavior

In more than half of the states, courts have ruled that employee handbooks form an implied contract between employer and employee. It's another limitation on employment at will in those states. Employers who fire a worker without following their handbook's policies on behavior and discipline could be sued for wrongful discharge. Many employers will have you sign an acknowledgment form that you've received a handbook. Once the acknowledgment form is signed, it's placed in your personnel file.

On the Job

Many of the laws that ban discrimination in hiring and firing also apply to discrimination on the job.

- The Age Discrimination in Employment Act applies to employees (and job seekers) who are over age 40. It requires that if a person over 40 is denied a promotion or job, the employer must be able to show why the younger person is more qualified. It also prevents employers from requiring employees to retire at a certain age. It's not advisable to ask how old any individual is during an interview to avoid any legal problems.

- The Americans with Disabilities Act prohibits an employer from discrimination on the basis of a worker's physical, mental, or medical disability. This includes discriminating against workers who have terminal cancer or are HIV positive. The law also requires employers to make reasonable adjustments to help a disabled worker function. Examples include making the break room wheelchair accessible and allowing the worker to miss work or come to work late, as long as it doesn't upset office operations. However, the ADA doesn't require remodeling or other changes that are very hard to make because of the office's layout or operations. Employees with alcohol and drug dependency issues are also protected under the ADA.

> If a business is remodeling or expanding its physical space, the changes must comply with ADA requirements. ADA compliance is also required if a business is sold.

- The Pregnancy Discrimination Act requires employers to treat a pregnant employee the same way they treat other employees, as long as she can do her job. The employer must allow her the same amount of sick leave and other time-off benefits that all other employees receive. But the employer can't force her to take a leave as long as she's able to work. The employer must also modify her job duties, if necessary, so that she can work as long as she wants to.

EMPLOYEE RIGHTS AND BENEFITS

Federal law also requires that employers provide certain benefits to their workers. For example, the Family Leave Act of 1991 requires that employers with 50 or more workers allow employees to take unpaid leave for any of the following reasons:

- pregnancy, childbirth, or care of a newborn child
- needs related to the adoption of a child
- care of an ill family member

Legal Brief 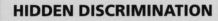 HIDDEN DISCRIMINATION

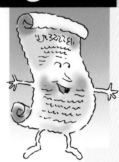

Discrimination can be hard to prove, because it's often not easy to spot. For example, a male and a female medical assistant both ask to go home 15 minutes early. The female's request is approved and the male's request is denied. That's not gender discrimination.

But if the employer grants most requests by women and denies most requests by men, then a case for discrimination could be made. In other words, it's generally a history or pattern of actions, not just a single act, that proves discrimination is taking place.

Even policies that treat employees equally can be discriminatory. That's because they sometimes affect different groups differently. For example, a requirement that all employees be able to lift heavy objects will be harder for women to meet, compared to men. Therefore, the policy would be a form of gender discrimination. Such policies are illegal, unless the employer can prove that they're necessary for doing the job.

The new parent does not need to be a woman to qualify for family leave. That's because letting a new mother take a leave while denying it to a new father would be discrimination based on gender.

Employees who work in small offices don't qualify for family leave, unless the employer permits it. However, employers that allow any kind of medical leave must allow maternity leave, too.

Workers' Compensation

Workers' compensation pays for employees' care if they suffer job-related injuries or develop some work-related disease. It makes no difference whether the employer or the employee was at fault. Workers' compensation also pays the employee for part of the wages she's losing while unable to work.

Almost every state requires employers to provide this protection for their employees. The employer either pays into a state workers' compensation fund or pays the premium for workers' compensation insurance for each employee.

If you're injured on the job, or become ill due to work-related causes, you must tell your employer immediately. If you're covered by workers' compensation, you can't sue your employer over the injury or disease, even if it was caused by the employer's actions.

Patient information regarding the workers' compensation claim should be maintained in a chart separate from the patient's regular chart. This is to help maintain patient confidentiality.

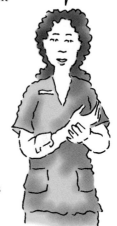

If you injure yourself at work, always notify your employer, even if it's just a small injury.

Unemployment Compensation

The Federal Unemployment Tax Act (FUTA) requires that employers also pay into a fund that makes temporary payments to workers who've lost their jobs through no fault of their own. Workers who quit are not entitled to this **unemployment compensation.** Neither are workers who were fired for cause or who go out on strike in a labor dispute.

Cause is not the same as *just cause.* **Cause** is misconduct that gives an employer a reason to fire an employee. In the law, **misconduct** is any violation of the employer's standards or rules. *Cause* can give an employer *just cause* to fire an employee. For example, making rude comments to patients may be the *cause* that gives an employer *just cause* to fire the employee. You'll learn more about this when you read about discipline later in the chapter.

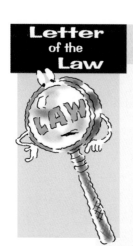

Letter of the Law

THE FAIR LABOR STANDARDS ACT

The Fair Labor Standards Act (FLSA) is an important law for medical offices, because they're often so busy that employees may work through lunch or stay beyond the end of the business day.

- The FLSA sets the standards for overtime pay when an hourly employee works more than 40 hours per week. With some exceptions, it applies to all full-time workers who earn less than $23,660 a year.
- Employers must pay hourly workers for 1.5 hours for each hour they work beyond 40 hours per week. It makes no difference whether the employer requires the overtime work or asks the employee to do it voluntarily.
- The rule does not apply to other workers who are classified as supervisors or as professional employees.

SEXUAL HARASSMENT

Sexual harassment is a common problem in the workplace. **Sexual harassment** is activity of a sexual nature that is unwanted by the person who comes into contact with it. It can range from off-color jokes and other verbal comments to pressure for sexual activity and actual sexual assault—such as patting and other forms of unwanted touching. Sexual harassment can occur between members of the opposite sex as well as between two members of the same sex.

Sexual harassment is a violation of Title VII of the Civil Rights Act of 1964. Most employers take sexual harassment very seriously. Many victims have successfully sued employers for allowing sexual harassment to continue in the workplace.

How an employer chooses to handle a person accused of sexual harassment typically depends on the nature of the harassment. Inappropriate looks and comments usually will result in counseling and a warning, if they were a first offense. Repeat offenses and more severe forms of harassment will be dealt with more severely. For example, any harassment that involves sexual assault or sexual battery will likely cause the harasser to be fired.

- **Sexual assault** is indecent sexual conduct that causes fear, shame, or mental suffering, or that involves threats or use of physical force against a person.

- **Sexual battery** is unwanted or forced touching of a person's sexual parts.

Sexual harassment is usually less about sex than it is about control or abuse of the victim by the harasser. For this reason, it can take two forms.

- *Quid pro quo.* This is a Latin term meaning "this for that." This form of harassment involves some kind of preferred treatment in exchange for sexual favors.

- **Hostile workplace.** This can include any behavior of a sexual nature that makes a workplace unpleasant for the person who feels harassed.

Quid Pro Quo Harassment

Quid pro quo sexual harassment takes place when someone in a dominant position over an employee (such as a physician) hints at or offers the employee job advancement or special considerations in return for sexual favors. The dominant person may be the office manager, the employee's direct supervisor, or even a physician. In addition, the "sexual favors" don't have to include intercourse. Even asking for a date can be *quid pro quo*

Ethics in Action

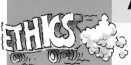

WORKPLACE RELATIONSHIPS: ARE THEY EVER OK?

The following types of romantic or sexual relationships are considered unethical in a medical setting, even if both parties consent and there's no sexual harassment involved:

- relationships between employees who work closely together; if neither wants to quit the job, one should ask to be assigned responsibilities that don't involve working with the other person.

- relationships between employee and supervisor; these are never acceptable because of the unequal power between the two people involved. It's unethical to continue both the sexual relationship and the supervisory one.

- relationships between employees and patients or their family members; these are unethical because they can affect medical decisionmaking and quality of care.

harassment if the employee feels pressure to accept because of the asker's position.

> Sexual harassment can occur no matter what the victim's or the harasser's gender.

Hostile Workplace

Sexual harassment also includes any kind of sexual activity that an employee finds offensive, even if it's not directed at the employee. For example, if other workers tell "dirty jokes" in the employee's presence or hang pictures or calendars of scantily clad figures where the employee can see them, a hostile workplace can result.

The key here is that the employee must make it clear to the offender that he or she is uncomfortable with the offender's behavior. If after knowing this, the offender continues the behavior, the employee has a good case for sexual harassment.

EMPLOYEE DISCIPLINE

Employers have a right to expect every employee to do his job well and not to behave in ways that interfere with office operations. At the same time, employees have a right to know what's expected of them. Poor communication in this area can lead to problems for both the employer and the employees. Poor performance, low morale, and even lawsuits can result.

Many employers try to prevent such problems by stating their expectations in an employee handbook or job description. The handbook may also state the possible consequences if an employee's performance or behavior doesn't meet the expected standards.

Discipline is an employer's policies and procedures for dealing with poor performance or behavior in the workplace. Most employers value their employees. They often have a lot of time and money invested in the employees' training and development. They don't want to fire their employees if it can be avoided.

Progressive Discipline

No employee is perfect, and employers realize this. Most use a process called progressive discipline to deal with performance and behavior that don't meet expectations. **Progressive discipline** is a series of increasingly severe steps that gives the employee a chance to improve poor conduct before being fired for it.

Progressive discipline benefits the employer, too. The focus on helping problem employees allows the employer to save its investment in those employees by not having to fire them. Progressive discipline also builds the employer's case for firing employees who do not improve. It strengthens the argument that they were fired for just cause and makes it harder for fired employees to win lawsuits for wrongful discharge.

Gross Misconduct

If an employee's poor performance or misbehavior is **gross** (extreme or severe), the progressive discipline steps can be skipped and she can be fired immediately. This is called **summary dismissal.** Here are some types of misconduct that are just cause for summary dismissal:

- committing a felony against a patient or a coworker
- refusal to obey a lawful and reasonable order
- gross neglect of job duties
- theft
- dishonesty
- gross incompetence that endangers patient care
- any misconduct that seriously threatens the health and safety of patients or coworkers, or the office's ability to function

Exhibits 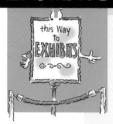 STEPS OF PROGRESSIVE DISCIPLINE

1. *Counseling.* The employer:
   - makes sure the employee understands what's required of him
   - discusses with the employee the poor performance or misconduct, how the problem can be corrected or avoided in the future, and offers help, if it's appropriate and possible
   - documents the meeting in the employee's personnel file even if it was a verbal warning
   - schedules follow-up evaluation meeting if necessary

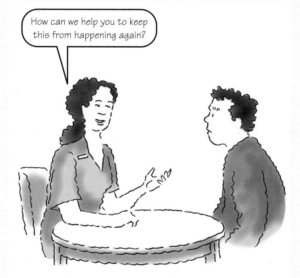

2. *Verbal warning.* If the problem continues, the employer:
   - reviews specifically what's expected of the employee
   - explains exactly how and why the employee is not meeting these requirements
   - makes another attempt to help the employee improve
   - describes possible consequences if the employee's performance or behavior doesn't improve
   - documents the meeting and the warning in the employee's file
   - schedules follow-up evaluation meeting if necessary

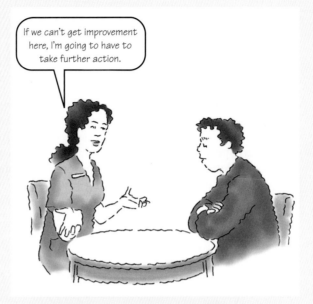

3. *Written warning.* If the problem continues, the employer:
   - tells the employee that his performance or behavior continues to be unsatisfactory
   - gives the employee a written statement that if the problem is not corrected, he will be put on probation
   - documents the meeting and places a copy of the warning in the employee's file
   - schedules follow-up evaluation meeting if necessary

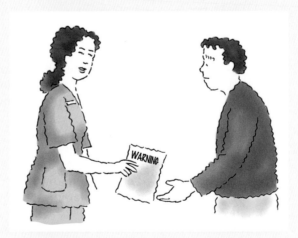

4. *Probation.* If the problem continues, the employer:
   - tells the employee that his performance or behavior continues to be unsatisfactory
   - gives the employee a written notice of probation that includes a statement of expectations and the possible consequences if they're not met
   - documents the meeting and places a copy of the probation notice in the employee's file
   - schedules follow-up evaluation meeting if necessary

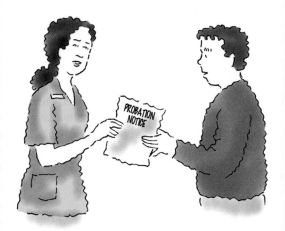

5. *Suspension.* If the problem continues, the employer:
   - tells the employee that his behavior continues to be unsatisfactory
   - sends the employee home, without pay, for up to five days
   - when the employee returns from the suspension, asks him to agree that there will be no further misbehavior
   - documents these actions in the employee's file

(This step applies only to misbehavior. In cases of poor performance, progressive discipline goes directly from step 4 to step 6.)

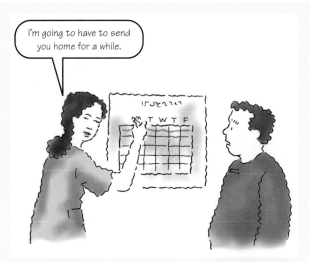

6. *Termination.* If the problem continues, the employer:
   - tells the employee that his performance or behavior has not satisfactorily improved and that he's still not meeting expectations and requirements
   - fires the employee
   - documents the action in the employee's file

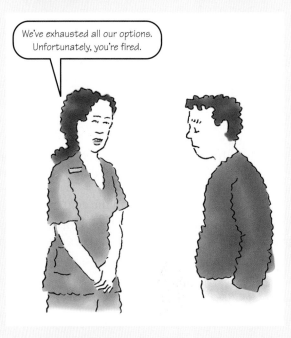

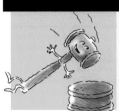

What's the Verdict?   CAN THEY FIRE ME?

A medical assistant who worked in the billing department of a group practice was almost always 15 minutes late to work in the morning. As a single mother, she had trouble getting the kids off to school and getting to work on time. She was counseled and warned by her supervisor, and even put on probation. When her behavior didn't change, she was fired.

She sued the employer for wrongful discharge and discrimination. She claimed that it was illegal to fire her, because her children made her late to work. She also claimed that her tardiness wasn't gross misconduct because, since she didn't have patient-care duties, it wasn't important to be there when the office opened each day.

The Verdict: The medical assistant lost her suit. The judge ruled that an employer has a right to decide the requirements for employment, including whether it's important to be at work on time. The employer's progressive discipline process had given her plenty of warning that she was not meeting those requirements and plenty of opportunity to improve. The judge also ruled that her tardiness *was* gross misconduct, because it was constant, which made it extreme misbehavior. Finally, the judge threw out her discrimination claim, noting that the fact that she had children was neither the direct nor the indirect reason she was fired.

Staying Safe in the Workplace

The Occupational Safety and Health Act of 1970 requires employers to provide a safe and healthy work environment for their employees. The law also created the Occupational Health and Safety Administration (OSHA) to write and enforce administrative rules for required standards of health and safety in the workplace.

OSHA's rules make both employers and employees responsible for workplace health and safety.

OSHA EMPLOYER REQUIREMENTS

Employers are required to:

- make all employees aware of OSHA health and safety requirements

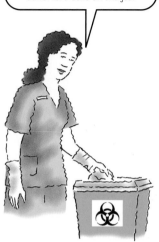

Remember: OSHA regulations are in place to keep you and your coworkers safe on the job.

- train employees to deal with workplace hazards safely.
- ensure that employees wear protective equipment when good safety practices require it
- keep certain records on workplace hazards and injuries
- report all workplace accidents to OSHA
- post a summary in the office of the previous year's work-related injuries and illnesses
- discipline employees for violating OSHA or employer safety rules
- avoid punishing employees who file complaints with OSHA about hazards in their workplace
- allow OSHA inspectors to conduct inspections of the workplace
- obtain the Material Safety Data Sheet (MSDS) from each chemical's manufacturer for every chemical housed in the facility

OSHA EMPLOYEE REQUIREMENTS

OSHA regulations require employees to:

- follow all OSHA health and safety standards that apply to their workplace
- obey all employer and OSHA safety rules
- use protective equipment when necessary
- report any hazardous conditions to their employer or to OSHA

OSHA INSPECTIONS

OSHA generally conducts inspections without advance notice. However, employers have a right to require OSHA officers to obtain a warrant before entering the workplace.

OSHA can't inspect all of the seven million work sites it regulates each year. It gives greatest attention to places with hazards that have a high risk of causing death or serious harm. OSHA officers can require an employer to correct hazards immediately or remove employees from the site.

Here are some other kinds of workplaces that are high on OSHA's list for inspection:

- employers who have had an incident that killed or hospitalized three or more employees

- employers whose employees have complained to OSHA about hazards or violations
- workplaces that may be hazardous according to reports from other people, government agencies, or the media
- follow-ups to check for correction of violations cited in previous inspections
- workplaces with a history of high illness or injury rates

Here's what happens in an OSHA inspection.

1. *The opening conference.* The OSHA inspector begins by explaining why the site was selected for inspection and what will happen next.

2. *The walk-around.* The inspector walks through the workplace looking for hazards that could lead to employee injury or illness and checking for compliance with OSHA rules about posted warnings. She may also interview employees. The employer has a right to accompany the inspector. Employees may also choose a worker to accompany the inspector.

3. *The closing conference.* The inspector meets with the employer and employee representatives to discuss her findings and the employer's choice of actions if violations have been found.

4. *The citation.* Within six months after the inspection, OSHA will send the employer a citation. It will list the violations, the proposed penalties, required corrective actions, and deadlines for making them.

5. *Appeals.* Employers have 15 days after receiving a citation to appeal it to the OSHA area director. This may result in reduced fines and a settlement agreement on how violations will be corrected. If the employer does not appeal, or if a settlement is not reached, the citation becomes final.

Penalties for violations can be severe—up to $7,000 per violation, and up to $70,000 per violation if it was deliberate or a repeat violation.

MEDICAL HAZARD REGULATIONS

The typical medical office contains many hazards that can put employees' health or safety at risk, if the proper precautions aren't followed. These hazards include:

- electrical and mechanical equipment
- chemicals, such as disinfectant sprays and lab chemicals
- blood and body fluids

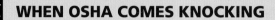

By the Book | WHEN OSHA COMES KNOCKING

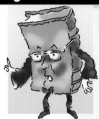

As a medical assistant, you may be at the reception desk when an OSHA inspector comes through the office door. Here's what to do—and what *not* to do!

- Ask the inspector for his OSHA identification, if he has not shown it. This is a reasonable request that won't cause any problems.

- Notify your supervisor that an OSHA inspector is in the office.

- Escort the inspector to the room where the opening conference will be held. Avoid taking him through any work areas, if you can.

- Remain with the inspector. Keep him company until your employer arrives.

- Don't allow the inspector to start the inspection without your employer's permission. In general, it's a good idea not to make the inspector's job more difficult. But your employer may want him to get a warrant first.

If you're asked to accompany the inspector on the walk-around:

- Follow the inspector. Don't attempt to guide him, hurry him, or otherwise interfere with his actions. Don't be afraid to ask questions.

- Take a digital or video camera with you, and a tape recorder to record his remarks. But first ask if he objects to this.

- Take a picture of anything the inspector takes a picture of. Also take pictures of things he points out to you.

- Remember that if the inspector becomes aware of any immediate danger during the walk-around, he's required to widen the scope of his inspection.

Finally, here are some general rules to follow, whether you go on the walk-around or the inspector decides to interview you:

- Treat the interview just as you would if asked to testify in court. Answer honestly, but only answer the questions asked. Don't provide any "extra" information.

- Don't argue with the inspector. Avoid making any comments not related to the inspection. Never criticize your employer or coworkers to the inspector.

- Be friendly, but don't try to be "best pals." Don't ask the inspector for a date, even for coffee, or make any comments about his appearance or clothing.
- The inspector is not allowed to accept anything as a gift—not even lunch—so don't make any offers.

The Hazard Communication Standard

OSHA requires that all employers have a written hazard communication program. This means that the employer must post a list of all hazards in the office in plain view. Employers must also compile a manual that provides information on each hazard, including how to protect against injury from it.

The hazards manual must contain a **Material Safety Data Sheet (MSDS)** for each chemical used in the office. It's the employer's responsibility to obtain the MSDS from each chemical's manufacturer. Here's what a chemical's MSDS tells about it:

- each ingredient in the product
- how to handle it safely and any protective equipment that must be worn
- any risks of the product catching on fire, exploding, or any other dangerous chemical reactions
- any risk of injury or illness if the chemical comes in contact with a person's skin or if someone breathes its fumes
- how to fight a fire resulting from the chemical
- how to treat someone who's been exposed to the chemical

OSHA rules require employees to read the MSDS before using a chemical and before cleaning it up in the event of a spill. Every chemical spill also requires an incident report that includes:

- the name of the chemical that was spilled
- the time, date, and place of the spill
- who was involved in the spill and how it was cleaned up

The Bloodborne Pathogen Standard

This OSHA standard is designed to protect health care workers from disease-causing organisms, such as HIV and hepatitis B, that can exist in patients' blood and other body fluids. Employers must post safety guidelines and have a written plan for controlling exposure to these organisms. Within the first 10 days of hire, the employer must also offer free hepatitis B vaccinations to any employee who is likely to be exposed to blood or body fluids.

Among other things, the regulations require employees to:

- cover all specimen containers with secure lids
- wear gloves and masks, if necessary, when handling patients' specimens
- dispose of used needles and other medical waste in proper hazardous waste containers
- immediately decontaminate surfaces on which body fluids have been spilled
- have a written procedure for routine daily cleaning and decontamination
- follow the hand-washing standards established by the Centers for Disease Control (CDC)

OSHA also requires employees to write incident reports if they're exposed to blood or body fluids, or if they accidentally stick themselves with needles. Employees as well as employers can be fined if they violate these OSHA rules.

CDC GUIDELINES

The Centers for Disease Control groups the tasks that medical office employees commonly perform into two categories.

- *Category I tasks.* These tasks expose the employee to contact with mucus membranes or skin contact that involves tissue, blood, or body fluids. Examples include throat cultures, pelvic exams, minor suturing, and phlebotomy. Gloves, goggles, and gowns are required when performing Category I tasks.

- *Category II tasks.* These tasks don't involve direct contact with blood, body fluids, or tissue. Protective equipment isn't required, but should still be worn since unplanned exposure might occur. Examples of Category II tasks include urinalysis, X-rays, injections, and ECGs.

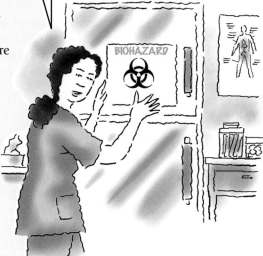

OSHA requires that biohazard warning labels be placed on anything that contains medical waste or infectious materials.

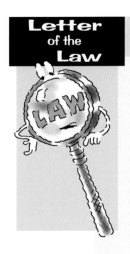

THE MEDICAL WASTE TRACKING ACT

The Medical Waste Tracking Act gives OSHA the authority to cite offices for unsafe or improper handling of hazardous medical wastes.

- Hazardous medical wastes include used needles; scalpels; grossly soiled examination table paper, gloves, and cotton swabs; blood products and other body fluids; body tissues; cultures; and vaccines.
- Needles and other sharps must be disposed of in approved puncture-proof containers.
- Other hazardous medical wastes must be disposed of in special leakproof, plastic biohazard bags.

CLIA AND THE JOINT COMMISSION

Congress passed the Clinical Laboratory Improvement Act (CLIA) in 1998 to set standards for laboratory testing.

- Labs that conduct tests on patient specimens must be inspected and certified by the Centers for Medicare and Medicaid Services (CMS).
- Labs must meet standards for test management, employee qualifications, quality control, and quality assurance.

The Joint Commission accredits laboratories, as well as all types of hospitals, managed-care organizations, and long-term care facilities. Many health care professionals expect that the Joint Commission will someday begin accrediting medical offices, too.

Medical offices already follow Joint Commission standards on what should be included in patients' medical records. Many medical offices also follow Joint Commission guidelines for identifying patients before giving them medications or drawing their blood. If the Joint Commission ever accredits medical offices, employees will have yet one more set of rules, regulations, and standards to follow.

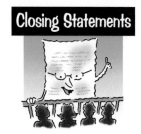

Closing Statements

- Employment at will governs the employer-employee relationship in most states. This allows an employer to fire an employee at any time, as long as the employer has a good reason for the termination and that reason is not an illegal one.

- It's illegal to fire someone because of race or national origin, religion, gender, age, disability, or pregnancy. In some states it's also illegal to fire a person because of family status, mental condition, physical appearance, or sexual orientation. It's illegal to treat an employee differently for these reasons, or to refuse to hire her. Collecting information from job applicants about these topics is illegal as well.

- Benefits that employers are required to provide employees include workers' compensation, unemployment compensation, and, in some cases, family leave. Family leave is time off for pregnancy, childbirth, adoption, or care of an ill family member. Employers who provide this benefit must allow both men and women to use it.

- Sexual harassment is unwanted sexual attention from another person. A person who receives such attention should make it clear to the harasser that the attention is unwanted. Employers will not tolerate sexual harassment in the workplace. Employees who sexually harass others may be severely disciplined or fired.

- Employers have the right to set standards for employee performance and behavior and to require employees to meet those standards. Employees have a right to know the standards they're expected to meet. Many employers provide this information in an employee handbook. When standards are not met, most employers use progressive discipline—a process of increasingly severe corrective actions—to allow employees the chance to improve, instead of firing them. In cases of extreme misconduct, the employee may be fired immediately.

- The Occupational Safety and Health Administration (OSHA) and the Centers for Disease Control (CDC) set standards for employee safety that employers and employees must obey. These requirements include standards for handling hazardous chemicals and medical wastes. Other requirements protect workers from disease-causing organisms that may be present in the blood, body fluids, and tissues of patients they treat.

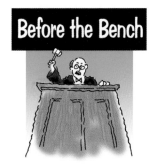

Before the Bench

Answer the following multiple-choice questions.

1. Which action does the doctrine of employment at will allow an employer to take legally?
   a. requiring an employee to retire when she reaches age 65
   b. requiring *all* employees to retire when they reach age 65
   c. laying off a worker who's no longer needed
   d. laying off a worker who has an employment contract

2. Which federal law does *not* protect a 50-year-old female employee from discrimination?
   a. the Fair Labor Standards Act
   b. the Civil Rights Act of 1964
   c. the Age Discrimination in Employment Act
   d. the Americans with Disabilities Act

3. Which question would be illegal to ask a job applicant during an interview?
   a. Can you work when the office is open on Saturdays?
   b. How many children do you have?
   c. Where did you get your training as a medical assistant?
   d. all of the above

4. All of the following can be required of a job applicant *except:*
   a. a psychological test.
   b. a credit check.
   c. a birth certificate.
   d. a physical examination.

5. Which action would be a wrongful discharge?
   a. firing an employee for joining a labor union
   b. firing an employee without just cause
   c. firing an employee for becoming pregnant
   d. all of the above

6. Which worker is entitled to unemployment compensation?
   a. a worker who quits
   b. a worker who goes on strike
   c. a worker who retires
   d. none of the above

7. Which of the following could be considered an example of sexual harassment?
   a. making an off-color joke at an employee meeting
   b. hanging a swimsuit calendar up in the office
   c. offering a salary increase in exchange for a sexual act
   d. all of the above

8. Which organization has the *most* influence over the health and safety of health care workers?
   a. the Occupational Safety and Health Administration (OSHA)
   b. the Centers for Disease Control (CDC)
   c. the Joint Commission
   d. the Equal Employment Opportunity Commission (EEOC)

9. What does OSHA require when a chemical is present in a medical office?
   a. that employees wear goggles and gloves when handling the chemical
   b. that employers install a fire extinguisher near where the chemical is stored
   c. that the employer have the chemical's Material Safety Data Sheet available for the employees to use
   d. that the employer notify OSHA before cleaning up any chemical spill

10. Which law helps create a healthier physical environment in a medical office?
    a. the Pregnancy Discrimination Act
    b. the Fair Labor Standards Act
    c. the Medical Waste Tracking Act
    d. all of the above

Chapter 9

PROFESSIONAL RELATIONSHIPS AND BEHAVIOR

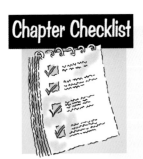

- Explain why it's important for medical assistants to follow the AAMA Code of Ethics

- Summarize the AMA Code of Ethics for physicians

- Discuss ethics as they pertain to the medical office

- Discuss how to abide by HIPAA guidelines as they pertain to drug representatives and other vendors

- Describe appropriate behavior with peers and vendors

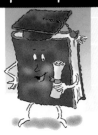

- Perform within legal and ethical boundaries (CAAHEP 3.c.2.b.)

- Maintain confidentiality at all times (ABHES 1.b.)

- Use appropriate guidelines when releasing records or information (ABHES 5.c.)

- Be cognizant of ethical boundaries (ABHES 1.d.)

In whatever medical setting you're employed, you'll be part of a team. You'll interact with other health care professionals and paraprofessionals who have different jobs, skills, and skill levels. It's also likely that you'll come into contact with other people who are not health care workers, including sales representatives for medical suppliers and drug companies. It's important that your dealings with all these people be as proper and professional as your relationships with patients.

Whether or not people are professionals, they are all individuals. Each individual has a unique personality. Not everyone's values and attitudes will complement your own. Nor will yours always match everyone else's. Differences will arise, and conflict may develop. For that reason, you'll read in this chapter about more than just professional and ethical behavior. You'll also learn how to establish the smooth office relationships that will help you work effectively as part of the team.

Behaving Professionally

First and foremost, professional behavior is proper behavior. "Proper" behavior is behavior that's appropriate for the following:

- *Your surroundings.* For example, loud and rowdy behavior is never appropriate in an office setting. Neither is gossiping about other employees.

In the medical office, remember that your behavior should always be "proper" and professional. Consider your surroundings, the situation, and the people involved before you act.

- *The situation or circumstances.* Remember that you're being paid to do a job. If you're conducting personal business, such as shopping on the Internet or making personal phone calls on office time, you are in effect stealing from your employer. That is not ethical behavior!

- *The person or people involved.* For example, it's highly improper to address the physician by his first name, unless he's asked you to do this. Otherwise, you should always refer to him as "the physician" or by his appropriate title and last name (for example, "Dr. Ortiz").

BEHAVING ETHICALLY

Proper behavior is also ethical behavior. In Chapter 1, you read about the American Association of Medical Assistants (AAMA) Code of Ethics. As you learned, this code outlines ethical behavior specifically for medical assistants. Topics covered in the code include protecting patient confidentiality and seeking to improve your knowledge and skills as a medical assistant. All medical assistants who gain the professional credential of Certified Medical Assistant (CMA) pledge to use the code as a guide to their professional behavior.

In addition to its Code of Ethics, the AAMA has created a creed that medical assistants should follow. A **creed** is a set of basic beliefs or principles to guide behavior. In Chapter 1, you learned that the AAMA Medical Assistant Creed focuses on integrity, fidelity, and other values that make up professional ethics. Following the guidelines presented in the AAMA Code of Ethics and adhering to the AAMA Medical Assistant Creed will enable you to act ethically in the situations you encounter in the medical office. You'll also be doing your part to protect the safety of patients and to protect the physician from possible legal action.

THE AMA CODE OF ETHICS

The physicians you'll work for also have a code of ethics to guide their behavior. The American Medical Association (AMA) Code of Ethics has been revised many times over many years.

The AMA's most recent code of ethics was written in 2004. It's a long document that is divided into the following sections:

- patient relationships
- professional conduct
- the physician's duty to society

As a medical assistant, you'll often be the link between physicians and patients. For example, you may be the first person the patient encounters when he calls or comes into the office. You may also represent the physician to the patient by carrying out assigned screening, treatment, or follow-up responsibilities.

You may be working for a DO, or doctor of osteopathy, instead of an MD. If that's the case, you should visit the website for the American Osteopathic Association at www.osteopathic.org to learn about the code of ethics for DOs as well.

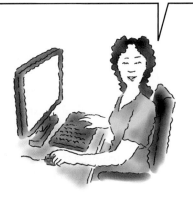

For these reasons, it's important to have a basic knowledge of the physician's ethical duties as they affect your job as a medical assistant. Many of them are guides that you should also follow, as the physician's representative. But in doing so, always remember the limits of your knowledge and training and the need to stay within your scope of practice.

Patient Care

The following standards from the AMA Code of Ethics for physicians apply to the physician's relationships with patients and to your relationships with patients as well.

- Consider first the well-being of your patient.
- Treat your patient with compassion and respect.
- Practice the science and art of medicine to the best of your ability (and within your scope of practice as a medical assistant).
- Make sure that you do not exploit your patient for any reason.
- Refrain from denying treatment to your patient because of a judgment based on discrimination.
- Maintain your patient's confidentiality. Exceptions to this must be taken very seriously.
- Recognize your professional limitations and be prepared to make referrals as appropriate.
- If you work in a practice or institution, place your professional duties and responsibilities to your patients above the commercial interests of the owners or others who work within these practices.
- Ensure security of storage, access, and utilization of information.

Professional Conduct

Some of the professional conduct requirements that the AMA Code of Ethics places on physicians can also apply to the medical assistants who work with them.

- Build a professional reputation based on integrity and ability.
- Recognize that your personal conduct may affect your reputation and that of your profession.
- Refrain from making comments that may needlessly damage the reputation of a colleague.
- Keep yourself up to date on relevant medical knowledge, codes of practice, and legal responsibilities.
- Report suspected unethical or unprofessional conduct by a colleague to the appropriate peer review body.

Medical assistants also have a responsibility to report suspected unethical or unprofessional conduct. However, their procedures for doing this differ from what a physician is ethically required to do. You'll learn more about reporting unethical or illegal conduct later in the chapter.

Dealing with Conflict

Years ago, a medical office typically consisted of a receptionist, the physician, and perhaps an office nurse. The work setting was a lot simpler. Good communication skills were less important than they are today.

With today's team approach to health care, many more people are involved in the delivery of services. This creates much more potential for **conflict,** or disagreement, resulting from people's differences. The more people who work in an office, the greater the potential for conflict. Conflict usually occurs in these situations:

- when one person's wants or needs are in conflict with another person's wants or needs
- when one person misunderstands another person's words or actions
- when one person is unable to understand or accept another person's beliefs or ideas
- when one person's expectations of another person are different from that person's expectations of himself

Conflict is especially common in the health care field. That's because it's an emotional and stressful business that involves the basic human needs for life and good health. Patients may be sick and frightened. Family members may feel helpless, angry, or sad. Keep this in mind if a patient or family member of a patient ever lashes out at you in anger or frustration. Most likely, the angry person is not upset at you, but is simply looking for somewhere to place her anxiety and fear.

Health care workers are often stressed by the physical and emotional demands of their work. The result can be conflict between a medical staff member and a patient or between staff members themselves.

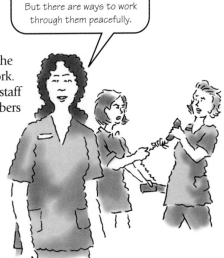

Conflicts are going to happen. But there are ways to work through them peacefully.

PERSONALITY AND BEHAVIOR

The ways people naturally respond to conflicts largely depend on their personalities. There are four main styles of behavior:

- passive behavior
- aggressive behavior

- assertive behavior
- passive-aggressive

Passive Personalities

Passive people will avoid conflict at all costs. They won't say what they really think about a situation because they fear that others might disagree. Putting other people's wants ahead of their own needs helps them to avoid conflict. For example, a passive person might not share her opinions about changes in office procedures during a team meeting because she does not want to get people upset.

Aggressive Personalities

Aggressive people are the exact opposite of passive people. In conflict situations they are confrontational. They try to "win" the conflict by dominating the other person. They seek to satisfy their own needs without considering the needs of others.

The reason aggressive behavior often works is because others may back down to avoid or defuse the situation. But aggressive behavior isn't effective in the long run. That's because those who are bullied by aggressive behavior, such as passive people, will often seek indirect ways to get even with the aggressor.

Assertive Behavior

Assertive people stand up for themselves while also showing concern for the needs of others. They directly express their views, wants, and needs in a non-threatening way. They deal with conflict by seeking agreement with others in ways that show respect for others as well as for themselves. Assertive people seek to solve problems in ways that don't damage relationships. You'll read more about assertive behavior shortly.

Passive-Aggressive Behavior

Passive-aggressive behavior combines traits from both passive and aggressive traits. Someone who behaves in a passive manner is generally reluctant to share opinions or true feelings in some situations. But problems can arise when some passive individuals secretly feel angry or resentful about a situation. They may see themselves as helpless victims of manipulation by others. They may even attempt to get revenge in indirect ways. For example, a passive person might not follow a required procedure as a way of "getting even" for another office situation.

COMMUNICATION IS KEY

Effective communication is key to preventing or resolving conflict between people. To be effective, communication must be clear and open. Also, both parties involved should have a positive attitude. The following sections describe several tips for communicating effectively.

Don't Assume

Breakdowns in communication can occur when you assume that you know what someone else is thinking. Assuming that others know what you know, think the way you think, or feel the way you feel is another block to effective communication. This behavior can lead to confusion and conflict. Instead, be open about what you're thinking and feeling, and ask others what they think and feel as well.

Have a Positive Attitude

Be friendly and engage others in conversation. Asking questions is a good way to open communication with your coworkers and patients. On the other hand, no one likes to listen to a whiner or complainer. You'll find that your communication with others will be more effective if you show a positive attitude.

Listen Actively

Be a good listener. Many people can express themselves clearly. But they often are not as good at listening. Failing to listen carefully to what another person says is probably the most common block to good communication. If you're not listening carefully to a patient, you may miss small but important details. These small omissions can have a detrimental effect upon the patient's care and the outcome of his treatment. Active listening requires that you give the speaker your undivided attention, even if you're busy and must temporarily stop doing other things. To listen attentively, pay attention to what the other person is saying, rather than using the time the other person is speaking to plan what you'll say in response.

Be Open-Minded

A judgmental attitude tells others that you don't really want to hear what they have to say. This can be a major block to effective communication. If a person thinks that you don't respect or believe what she's telling you, she'll probably stop talking. You reveal a judgmental attitude with your body language, facial expressions, or comments you make.

Being open-minded involves considering points of view other than your own. To communicate effectively, avoid making any judgments until you have all the facts. Convey an open-minded attitude by giving the other person enough time to explain her thoughts, feelings, or concerns without interrupting. Maintain a calm manner, and make sure your body language and facial expressions communicate your desire to be open-minded about the situation. For example, you might turn your body toward the person speaking and uncross your arms to display "open" body language. Additionally, you might convey concern or attentiveness in your facial expressions. Doing so will help keep the lines of communication open.

When you want a coworker to know that you're welcome to new ideas, let your body do the talking! Relax your arms at your sides and maintain a pleasant, calm facial expression while the other person is speaking.

DEALING WITH CONFLICT

No matter how open-minded you are, no matter how positive or how good a listener you are, you'll still encounter conflict. There's no avoiding it, especially in a busy, high-stress, and pressure-filled medical office. You might find yourself in conflict with your supervisor, a physician, a nurse, or another coworker. How you deal with it can directly affect your work as a member of the health care team.

There are several methods for resolving conflicts. Some work well in certain situations. Others are not truly solutions at all, but are merely temporary fixes. Here's a list of the most common methods of conflict resolution. Keep in mind that not every method is necessarily appropriate in every situation.

Accommodation

Accommodation is adapting or adjusting to something. In a conflict situation, it means simply giving in to the other person. Although this can preserve the relationship between the two people, it requires one of them to give up what he needs or wants. So, this approach to solving the conflict leaves one party the winner and the other feeling like the loser. For this reason, it's usually not the best or permanent solution for a conflict.

Avoidance

Avoidance is the act of withdrawing or ignoring a situation. Avoidance is also not a permanent solution to conflict. It only postpones the settlement of the issue. But, sometimes, it's an effective temporary solution. For example, during a heated argument, it might be best just to walk away from the discussion. This gives both parties time to calm down before getting back together to try and find a solution.

Compromise

Compromise is a process in which each party in a dispute gives up some of her demands to achieve other demands. This method for resolving conflict makes each side partly a winner and partly a loser. It may not provide a permanent settlement because each party is only partly satisfied. For this reason, the settlement of conflicts by compromise is often only temporary. The unmet demands of either side may arise again at a later time.

Competition

Competition is a method for settling conflicts in which the stronger party forces a solution on the other party. It generally only works in an emergency, when there isn't time for discussion, or when all other strategies have failed.

Collaboration

Collaboration is a process in which each party in a conflict cooperates with the other party until they can both agree upon a solution. It's the only strategy for resolving conflicts that provides a "win" for both sides.

Workplace Relationships

As a medical assistant, you'll be dealing with a variety of people every day. They include supervisors, coworkers, physicians, vendors, and, of course, patients. (A **vendor** is a seller of something, such as a drug company or a company that sells medical supplies.) Doing your job effectively will require assertive behavior in your dealings with all these people. This is especially true in situations that involve conflict and matters of ethics or law.

BEING ASSERTIVE

It's likely that you'll have to deal with others who do not share your values and ethical standards. In fact, there may be times when you may feel pressured to do something that is unethical or even illegal. It's important for you to be assertive in such situations. Some strategies you can use to develop an assertive style of behavior begin on page 222.

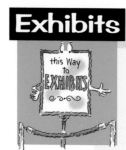

Exhibits

THE CONFLICT RESOLUTION PROCESS

It's not professional behavior to go running to your supervisor whenever you have a conflict with a coworker. It's also unprofessional to get involved in a public argument or confrontation. Here's a step-by-step strategy for resolving conflicts in a professional manner:

1. If a conflict arises with a coworker, speak to her privately about it. Thank her in advance for giving you her time.

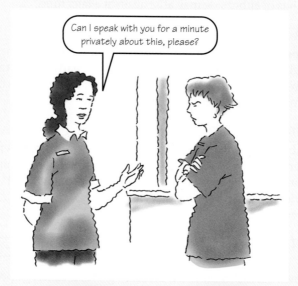

2. Focus on the specific area of conflict during your conversation. Avoid talking about your personal feelings to the person or telling her how she should be acting or feeling.

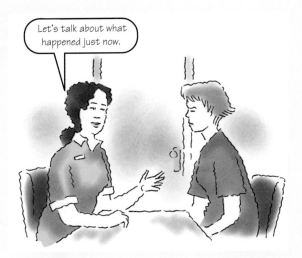

3. Take responsibility for your emotions by expressing how you feel rather than accusing her for your feelings. For example, instead of saying, "You really upset me with what you said," say, "I feel upset by what you said."

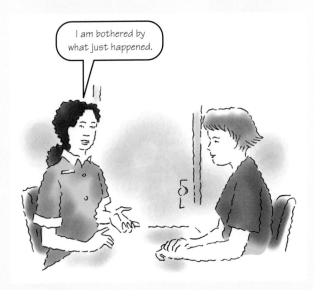

4. Allow the other person to explain her side, even if it's hurtful or unpleasant to hear. Perhaps the conflict results from a misunderstanding of something that was done or said. If so, apologize for the misunderstanding.

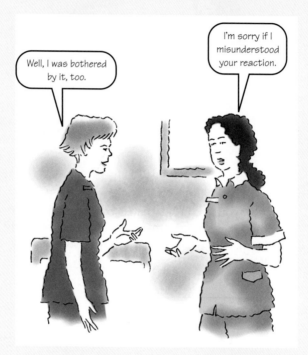

5. Ask the other person for her ideas about how the conflict might be resolved. Her suggestions may provide a better solution than your own.

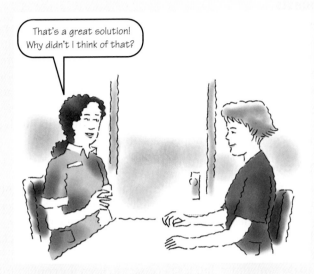

6. Not all conflicts can be resolved. Sometimes, you just have to "agree to disagree" on certain things and focus on the things you have in common. However, if the conflict affects patient care, it can't be allowed to continue. In such a case, you and the coworker should go together to your supervisor.

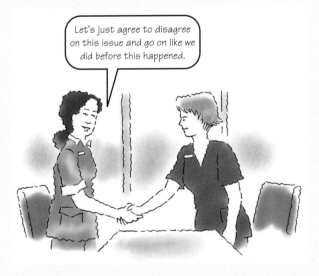

Making Requests

Asking for what you want in a direct manner is an important part of behaving assertively. This includes being able to ask for help when you need it. It also includes making it clear to others what you expect of them. Finally, it involves trusting others to respond to your requests in an assertive way. This may sometimes mean that you won't get the response you desire. You must not overreact to such responses if you want your communication with the person to continue in an honest, assertive way.

Recognizing Provocations

When conflict arises, some people may try to "win" by attempting to bully or humiliate you. For example, an aggressive coworker or a patient who feels helpless may lash out at you with a personal attack. Behaving assertively requires that you ignore such tactics and focus on solving the problem instead. This can be hard to do sometimes. But it's necessary to keep the conflict from increasing and possibly damaging important relationships.

Setting Limits

The ability to set limits is a basic part of assertive behavior. It's a skill that's necessary to avoid feeling overwhelmed, angry, and taken advantage of by other people whose wants and needs conflict with our own. Setting limits does not mean that you stop saying "yes" to requests. But it *does* mean being honest when those requests will cause you difficulty in meeting them.

Being Persistent

Another important part of being assertive is being persistent—that is, refusing to give up—in making sure that your rights are respected. Once you've said "no" or set some other kind of limit, people often will try to talk you into changing your mind. They may try to make you feel guilty or wrong by questioning your reasons. In such cases, simply continue to repeat your decision, without becoming aggressive or defensive. This technique of calmly repeating your decision is called the "broken record" response. It will help you stand firm against even the most aggressive person without increasing the level of conflict.

The broken record technique may be especially helpful if you ever have to deal with a drug-seeking or otherwise persistent patient. You may be the one who has to tell the patient that the physician is not going to renew her prescription. Once the drug-seeking patient has been told this, she may try to convince you over and over why she needs the medication. By repeating your

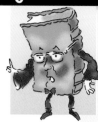

By the Book   RESPONDING ASSERTIVELY

Here are some strategies for assertive behavior in setting limits.

- Decide what or how much you're willing to do in the situation or to meet the request.
- If you need time to think about it, it's appropriate to say so as long as you get back to the other person within the time you say you will. Something like "I need some time to think about this. Can I get back to you by the end of the day?" would be an appropriate way to communicate your need to think more about the situation.
- Your response does not always have to be "yes" or "no." In many cases you may be able to offer to meet a request partially instead.
- It's more difficult to say "no" if you fear that the other person might not agree with your reasons for doing so. You can avoid this "guilt trap" by not providing specific reasons for your decision.

"No" response like a broken record, you may find it easier to remain calm until the patient stops asking.

ASSERTIVENESS WITH EMPLOYERS

It's just as important to be assertive with supervisors as it is with coworkers. We often have a tendency to do what we are told when communicating with supervisors. However, as a health care professional, you may find yourself in a situation where a supervisor does not share or understand your profession and its ethical standards. It's important to be assertive in maintaining those standards when they are threatened by the requests or demands of others.

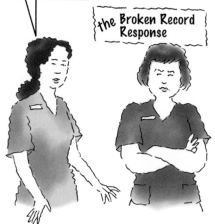

ASSERTIVENESS WITH VENDORS

You may come into contact with different types of vendors in your work as a medi-

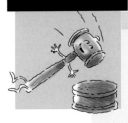

What's the Verdict?

IF THE PHYSICIAN ASKS YOU TO DO SOMETHING UNETHICAL

The physician asks you to bill a patient's insurance for services that were not provided, or that were provided at a lower cost. You've learned about upcoding, and you know it's an unethical practice. What should you do in this situation?

The Verdict: First, approach the physician privately and ask him if he's aware that what he's asked you to do is illegal (or unethical). If he insists, you should take the matter to your supervisor. If that doesn't work, your last resort is to report the situation to the appropriate authority. For example, upcoding would be reported to the insurance company. Violations of professional ethics would be reported to the appropriate professional body, such as the AMA or state licensing board.

These actions should be last resorts because they could cost you your job. When reporting something illegal, however, you'd be protected by whistleblower law. The principle of *qui tam* that you read about in Chapter 5 would apply. So if you were to be fired, you'd have a case for wrongful termination.

It's important to understand that going along with an illegal act makes you an accessory to the crime. You can be punished along with the person who asked you to do it.

cal assistant. Salespeople will visit the office with samples of medications and medical supplies for the physician. In the past, salespeople for medical supply companies and drug companies mingled freely with medical office workers. Now, because of HIPAA's strict requirements on patient confidentiality, vendors must be restricted from areas in which patients' charts are present. Although the salespeople should be aware of your office's policy, you may need to remind them from time to time to be sure that patients' private information is protected.

Other vendors may also come into contact with private information about patients. These vendors include outside billing companies, companies who convert paper charts to electronic records, and medical office cleaning companies. These vendors must also comply with HIPAA's confidentiality requirements to ensure patient privacy. If you're concerned that HIPAA's confidentiality rules are violated at any time, you should assert your-self and let your supervisor know immediately.

Common Workplace Conflicts

In your work as a medical assistant, you'll deal with patients and coworkers on a daily basis. In this chapter you've learned about personality types and effective communication tech-niques for dealing with them. Now, here are some common types of situations that you're likely to encounter.

CONFLICTS WITH PATIENTS

A common problem that you're likely to face in a medical office is responding to angry or critical patients. Their hostility toward you may very well be unfair and undeserved. And it's easy to get caught up in that emotion and defend yourself by responding in the same way. But to keep the situation from worsening, it's important to keep in mind that their hostility is probably inten-sified by the stresses they're experiencing.

Most patients are ill, and some are seriously ill. They may be feeling helpless and dependent on the office's employees. When they experience extended waiting times, their suffering and anxiety may cause them to lash out inappropriately. It's important to understand that in most cases their frustration is mainly about being ill and not because of personal grievances against you.

As you've read in earlier chapters, the key to dealing with patients is to show empathy and understanding. Here are some ways to deal with angry patients by showing both understand-ing and assertiveness:

- agreeing with the patient
- turning criticism into helpful feedback
- standing up for yourself

I Agree!

Agreeing with the patient shows understanding and empathy. For example, if a patient reacts with anger at the cost of a treat-ment, you might say, "You're right, this treatment is expensive. Would you be interested in looking at some payment options we have available?" This response shows that you understand the patient's concern. It also allows you to determine if the cost of treatment is the real source of his anger.

Room for Improvement

Another way you can display understanding and assertiveness is by turning criticism into feedback. For example, if a patient complains that office workers are uncaring, ask, "What specifically upset you?" His response could be useful for improving the way the office operates. Or it could show a need for better and clearer communication.

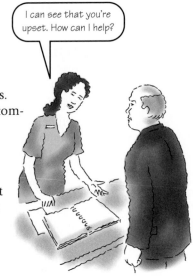

I can see that you're upset. How can I help?

Stand Up for Yourself

Sometimes a patient will remain aggressive despite your efforts to calm the situation. In that case, you'll need to set limits without becoming aggressive yourself. Calmly say something like, "I want to hear your point of view, but I don't want to be screamed at. When you're ready to talk without yelling and swearing, I'll listen."

SEXUAL HARASSMENT

Sexual harassment is another common source of workplace conflict. You read about the legal aspects of sexual harassment in Chapter 8.

If you receive unwanted sexual attention from a coworker, you should quietly and privately make your feelings known to that person. This can be difficult if the harasser is someone in a position of authority, such as a supervisor. You may fear unpleasant consequences if you resist. But it's important that you clearly communicate that the attention is unwanted.

If the harassment continues after you've made your feelings known, you should report it to your supervisor. (If the incident involved an assault, it should be reported immediately.) If your supervisor is the harasser, you should report it to that person's supervisor. As a last resort, or if the harassment continues after you've reported it, you can file a complaint with the Equal Employment Opportunity Commission (EEOC).

A FINAL WORD ON WORKPLACE RELATIONSHIPS

There will be times that you'll observe unethical, illegal, or other improper behavior by your coworkers, without being the victim or target of it.

- You might overhear a coworker using foul language with a patient.

- You might witness a coworker not treating an older adult patient with dignity and respect.

- You might become aware that a coworker is stealing money, supplies, or drugs from the office.

It's important that you handle such situations properly and professionally.

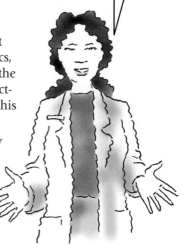

Addressing a coworker's improper behavior is never easy. If the offense isn't serious, speak with your coworker privately before reporting the behavior to a supervisor.

- When the behavior is improper but does not involve a serious breach of professional ethics, the best course is usually a private talk with the person using the communication and conflict-handling strategies you've learned about in this chapter.

- Misbehavior that involves illegal or seriously unethical conduct must be reported to your employer. Patient abuse and theft would fall into this category. In most cases, your immediate supervisor is the person to turn to.

Closing Statements

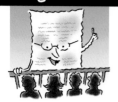

- Proper professional behavior should be legal, ethical, and appropriate to the surroundings, situation, and persons involved.

- The AAMA Code of Ethics provides a basic guide to proper behavior for medical assistants. Parts of the AMA Code of Ethics for physicians are also appropriate in situations in which the medical assistant is acting as the physician's representative.

- Good communication skills are needed to deal with conflicts that occur in the normal daily operations of a medical office.

- Conflicts will naturally arise due to the stressful nature of a medical office and to personality differences among its employees.

- People generally exhibit three main types of behaviors, which are shaped by their personalities: passive behaviors, aggressive behaviors, and assertive behaviors.

- Behaving assertively is the best way to resolve conflict fairly. Assertive behavior requires being direct without being aggressive. It also involves ignoring provocations, setting limits, and being persistent in your efforts to foster respect for yourself, for your coworkers, and for their differences.

- Conflicts with patients are a common problem in a medical office. Good communication and assertive behavior techniques can reduce this problem. Sexual harassment is another common problem that can be handled in this manner.

- Other problems and conflicts with coworkers should also be resolved by the parties themselves when possible, unless illegal or unethical behavior is involved. Illegal behavior and serious breaches of ethics must be reported to supervisors.

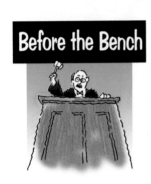

Before the Bench

Answer the following multiple-choice questions.

1. A good guide to proper behavior for medical assistants can be found in
   a. the AAMA Code of Ethics.
   b. the AAMA Creed.
   c. the AMA Code of Ethics.
   d. all of the above

2. Which value is common to the AAMA Code of Ethics, the AMA Code of Ethics, and the AAMA Creed?
   a. protecting patient confidentiality
   b. serving the well-being of society
   c. self-improvement
   d. all of the above

3. Why is conflict more common in health care than in many other fields?
   a. Physicians are hard to get along with.
   b. Health care is delivered by a team.
   c. The emotional and physical stresses are high.
   d. The competition for new patients is intense.

4. What is a good strategy for getting along in a medical office?
   a. Avoid conflict at all costs.
   b. Stand up for yourself, but respect other people's needs.
   c. Complain about all injustices.
   d. Always put other people's needs ahead of your own.

5. Which person is *most* likely to be a resentful and unhappy worker?
   a. someone with a passive personality
   b. someone with a competitive personality
   c. someone with an aggressive personality
   d. someone with an assertive personality

6. Which person is *least* likely to be a resentful and unhappy worker?
   a. someone with a passive personality
   b. someone with a competitive personality
   c. someone with an aggressive personality
   d. someone with an assertive personality

7. The key to settling conflicts in the medical office is
   a. standing up for your beliefs.
   b. being committed to "winning" the conflict.
   c. practicing effective communication skills.
   d. having a positive attitude.

8. The best and most permanent solutions to conflicts are achieved through
   a. accommodation.
   b. compromise.
   c. collaboration.
   d. all of the above

9. Which of the following is *not* an assertive behavior?
   a. giving up your rights for the good of others
   b. requesting help when you think you need it
   c. setting limits on what you're willing to do
   d. avoiding or ignoring the provocations of others

10. If you're asked to do something illegal, you should
    a. make sure the requester knows that it's illegal.
    b. refuse to grant the request.
    c. notify your supervisor if the requester pushes the matter.
    d. all of the above

Chapter 10

BIOETHICS

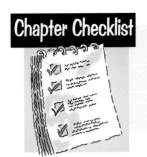

Chapter Checklist

- Explain what an advance directive is and the benefits of having one

- List and describe the stages of grief

- Explain why bioethical issues need to be addressed and provide six examples of current bioethical issues

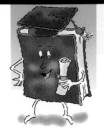

Chapter Competencies

- Demonstrate knowledge of federal and state health-care legislation and regulations (CAAHEP 3.c.2.f.)

- Be cognizant of ethical boundaries (ABHES 1.d.)

Medical science and the practice of medicine have made tremendous advances in recent years. It's now possible to do things to and with the human body that could hardly be imagined 50 years ago. People who have died are kept "alive" on machines. Children are conceived outside their mother's body. Women are pregnant with babies that aren't their own. People have organs in their bodies that used to belong to someone else or even to an animal!

Medicine has reached the point that it can affect life in ways that seem unnatural to some people. Some question whether medicine has gone too far. They ask, "Just because we *can* do something, does that mean that we *should* be doing it?"

Answering such questions involves a kind of ethics called bioethics. Bioethics deals with what's "right" when issues of life and death can be decided by advances in medical science. In this chapter you'll read about bioethical issues that you're likely to encounter in a medical office.

Death and Dying

When is someone dead? This may seem like a simple question, but defining when life ends is nearly as controversial as defining when it begins.

Until fairly recently, death occurred when a person's heart stopped. But today, drugs allow physicians to keep a heart working when it will no longer beat on its own. These and other artificial means that continue a person's vital functions are known as **life support.** They are the reason why the legal definition of death now includes **brain death.** People are now legally dead when *either* their brain or their heart stops working.

Some people don't accept the idea of brain death. They believe that a person is alive as long as his heart is beating. They claim that discontinuing life support is the same as killing a patient.

Other people reply that you can't "kill" someone who has no brain activity. That's because he's dead already. They argue that without the brain death standard, life support could keep a body "alive" forever. These distinctions can be confusing, and it's not uncommon to wonder, "when is someone really dead?" Unfortunately, there is no easy answer to this question, but studying bioethics can help you see the different sides of issues surrounding life and death.

You'll probably never have to deal with these issues in a clinical setting as they mainly affect hospital and nursing home employees. But many medical offices do have patients who are **terminally ill.** This means that a person has a condition from which he's expected to die soon. Treating such patients involves a set of legal and ethical issues that can be as controversial as determining when a patient is dead.

TERMINALLY ILL PATIENTS

Treating someone who's in the final stages of a terminal disease can require some of the most morally difficult decisions in health care. A **terminal disease** is a disease for which there is no reliable cure and that will eventually kill the patient.

Every person has a right to life. But prolonging a life that is going to end soon can drain a family's finances and extend the patient's pain and suffering. Patients may seek guidance from the physician or others on the "right" thing to do in such situations.

The decision to live or die belongs to the patient, if she's competent to make it. Judging a patient's competence in such cases depends on several things.

- Does the patient truly understand the situation and the issues involved?
- Is the patient able to reason, based on the information she's been given?
- Is the patient able to communicate a choice?

> From a physician's perspective regarding treatment being administered, there's no ethical difference between stopping treatment that is keeping a person alive and withholding such treatment.

If the patient is not competent, then the physician must make all treatment decisions, unless there's someone who's legally empowered to speak for the patient. (You'll learn more about this subject shortly, when you read about advanced directives.) One of two ethical principles will guide the physician in making this decision.

1. *Substituted judgment test.* What decision would the patient probably make if she were able to make the decision?

2. *Best interest standard.* What's best for the patient under the circumstances?

If the answer in both cases is the same, the physician's course of action is clear. But when these two principles are at odds, an ethical dilemma can result. Does the physician do what's medically best for the patient under the circumstances? Or does he do something else in case the patient might not have made the same choice as the physician?

The Right to Die

In general, patients have the right to refuse treatment that would prolong their life. The health care provider has two duties in this situation:

- to make sure the patient understands that the decision will probably end her life; think of this as a type of informed consent. This option should always be presented during informed consent as the option to "do nothing."
- to provide only care that treats the patient's pain and allows her to be as comfortable as possible; this is known as **palliative care.** However, the patient has the right to refuse even this level of care.

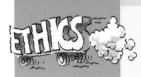

Ethics in Action — HEROIC MEASURES

Terminally ill patients sometimes will turn to "miracle cures" in a desperate effort to save their own lives. Physicians are not required to provide such treatments if they offer no medical benefit. If a patient insists, and the physician feels that providing the treatment is unethical, he must arrange to transfer the patient to another provider.

If a physician objects on moral or ethical grounds to the patient's decision to die, he must refer her to another provider who will follow her wishes for treatment.

Euthanasia

Euthanasia is purposely ending the life of someone who is suffering. It's also known as mercy killing. Although in Greek euthanasia means "good death," it's another troubling legal and ethical issue.

Under the law, killing a person is murder, even if that person is suffering and would die soon anyway. But what if such a person asks someone to help him take his own life? This form of euthanasia is called assisted suicide.

In general, physician-assisted suicide is said to occur when a physician prescribes a fatal dose of medication that the patient can take when she feels the time is right. Typically, the patients who seek to find a physician who would be willing to participate in this type of euthanasia are patients who have seriously debilitative and/or terminal diseases such as amyotrophic lateral sclerosis (ALS) (also known as Lou Gehrig's disease).

Physician-assisted suicide remains controversial. One physician who injected a patient with a fatal drug at the patient's request was convicted of murder and sent to prison. Supporters argue that it's part of a patient's right to die; critics reply that letting a patient choose death is one thing, but that helping him do it is wrong. The American Medical Association (AMA) opposes assisted suicide as contrary to the physician's duty as a healer.

ADVANCE DIRECTIVES

Another, less controversial, way that law and medicine have dealt with right-to-die issues is by allowing advance directives. An **advance directive** is a written statement of a patient's treatment wishes if the patient is not able to state his wishes at the time. There are three kinds of advance directives that can affect a patient's treatment:

- a living will
- a durable power of attorney, often referred to as a POA
- a health care proxy

A fourth type of advance directive is the organ donor directive. You'll learn more about this when you read about organ donation later in the chapter.

The Living Will

A **living will** is a document the patient writes in advance that gives the physician instructions about the patient's treatment wishes if the patient is not able to make her wishes known at the time. A living will may include any or all of the following information:

- descriptions of conditions under which the patient does not want to be treated, or to have current treatment continued—for example, coma, brain death, or some terminal condition
- specific treatments the patient does not want started or wants suspended—such as feeding tubes, machines that breathe for the patient, and other measures that don't treat the condition but merely delay death
- extraordinary measures—such as emergency surgery or measures to restart the heart—that the patient does not want used

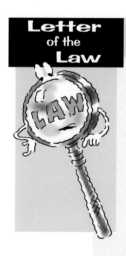

Letter of the Law

THE PATIENT SELF-DETERMINATION ACT

The Patient Self-Determination Act of 1990 requires physicians to give patients written information about their rights under the laws in their state to make medical decisions and to prepare advance directives. The act also requires physicians to do the following:

- document in the patient's chart whether he has provided an advance directive
- avoid discrimination against a patient based on whether he has an advance directive
- obey all state laws regarding advance directives
- educate staff about advance directives

The patient may also state her wishes about organ donation or an autopsy in a living will. A copy of a patient's living will should be placed in her office medical record. It's important that the family members are also aware of the patient's wishes because many times in emergency situations, the patient is not able to communicate her wishes. In these situations, it will be up to the family to make difficult health care decisions. When the family members know the patient's wishes, they may find it easier to make decisions regarding her health care.

AUTOPSIES

An autopsy is an examination of a body's organs and tissues to determine what caused a person's death. The law requires an autopsy when foul play is suspected. An autopsy also may be required if the death was suspicious for other reasons—for example, a young, seemingly healthy person dies unexpectedly for unknown reasons.

When a patient dies, the physician may ask the patient's family to consent to an autopsy to determine the exact cause of death. Sometimes families will ask for an autopsy, seeking comfort in the reassurance that their loved one could not have been saved. But public attitudes about autopsies are changing, and consent for such autopsies is declining. Family members may deny an autopsy for the following reasons.

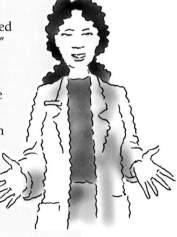

Remember that family members can't deny an autopsy if the law requires one for reasons of suspected foul play.

- They feel that their loved one already suffered enough and don't want his body "damaged" further after he's gone.
- They fear that an autopsy would prevent or interfere with the viewing of the body at the funeral.
- They may believe that modern medicine can provide enough information about the cause of death without an autopsy.

Health care providers may not agree with these views about autopsies, but they must be sensitive to the family's beliefs and emotions.

The Durable Power of Attorney

A **durable power of attorney** is a document a patient may sign that names another person to make decisions for the patient if the patient is not able to make them for himself.

- The durable power of attorney takes effect if the patient is not conscious or if he becomes incompetent for other reasons.
- The patient may place limits in the document on the responsibilities of the person he names.
- The document may also give instructions about the patient's wishes in certain situations.

If an office patient has a durable power of attorney, a copy of it should be made and placed in his medical record. A patient may revoke or change a durable power of attorney at any time. It's the patient's responsibility to inform the family members as to who he has chosen to have durable power of attorney.

> A health care proxy is sometimes known as a power of attorney for health care.

The Health Care Proxy

A **health care proxy** is like a durable power of attorney, except that it applies only to health care. The person the patient names in a health care proxy has authority to make only health decisions for the patient.

- The patient must be in a position or state of mind where he is unable to make decisions for himself before the health care proxy takes effect.
- The document may also include the patient's wishes about certain care or treatments that should be allowed or rejected.
- A health care proxy may also put other limits on the authority of the person named to make decisions for the patient.

Like living wills and durable powers of attorney, a copy of a patient's health care proxy should be kept in his office chart.

GRIEF AND GRIEVING

As a medical assistant, you may have contact with dying patients. Patients who have been diagnosed with a terminal disease often experience deep grief. Grief is a normal human reaction to loss—whether it's the loss of a job, a marriage, a loved one, or of one's own life.

Medical office employees can be a good source of support for such patients. But it's important to understand grief and the grieving process so that your efforts will be helpful and not resented by the patient or his family.

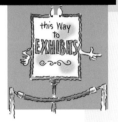

Ethics in Action
WHEN A LIVING WILL AND POWER OF ATTORNEY CONFLICT

Sometimes a patient will have a living will and also will have given someone power of attorney (POA). In general the person with the POA should follow the wishes the patient expressed in the living will. However, changing circumstances can bring those wishes into question. The physician is required to follow the directions of the patient's representative in such cases. This ethical requirement is based on the principle of substituted judgment.

Exhibits
THE GRIEVING PROCESS

Authorities on death and dying have identified five steps or stages in the process of grieving a loss. They may not always occur in this exact order. But a terminally ill patient must experience them all before coming to terms with his death.

Stage 1: *Denial.* The patient refuses to believe that the diagnosis is correct. This stage is usually very temporary. Few terminally ill patients continue to deny their condition until their death.

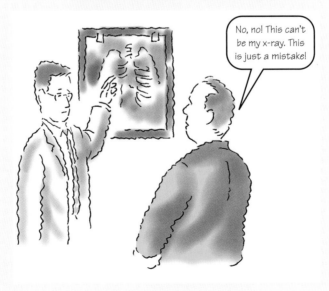

Stage 2: *Anger.* When the patient can no longer deny his illness, he may then become angry and resentful at his loss of control over his body and life. He may lash out at others with blame or withdraw into an angry silence.

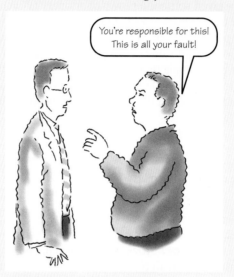

Stage 3: *Bargaining.* A terminally ill person will often offer to change some behavior if death can be avoided or postponed. Family members may feel guilt or responsibility for the patient's death.

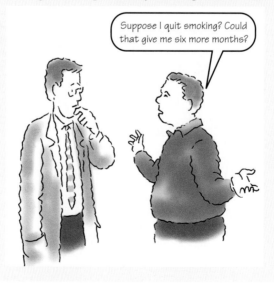

Stage 4: *Sadness.* The patient will become depressed
and feel that his situation is hopeless. He may
cry frequently and may not want to continue
daily activities. If this stage goes on for long,
he should be encouraged to seek help from a
mental health professional.

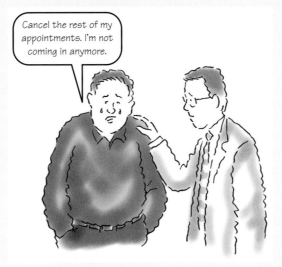

Stage 5: *Acceptance.* The terminally ill patient finally
accepts his loss. This might be shown by writing a
will or making other arrangements for his death.

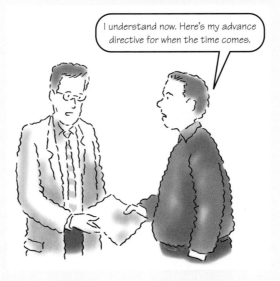

By the Book   PROVIDING SUPPORT

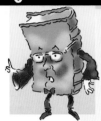

As a medical assistant, you're in a good position to provide support to a terminally ill patient. Here are some points to keep in mind.

- Make yourself available to talk, but don't force a conversation. Say something like, "You look worried. Do you feel like talking?" If the patient says "no," let her know that you're available if she ever does want to talk.

- When talking with the patient, don't appear rushed. Sit down, relax, and act ready to listen. If the patient is angry or resentful, don't respond in the same way. Encourage the patient to continue by saying things like, "What do you mean?" or "Go on; I understand."

- Don't try to change the subject if you become uncomfortable. Instead, admit your discomfort. Don't be afraid to describe your own feelings. It's okay to say "I find this difficult to talk about." But encourage the patient to keep talking.

- Don't offer advice, even if the patient asks for it. Instead, listen to the patient, and then suggest that the patient may want to discuss the concerns with a family member or the physician. And don't ever offer medical advice or opinions. Suggest that the patient direct such questions to the physician or nurse.

- Don't be afraid to laugh with the patient, but don't try to cheer her up with your own jokes. Remember that grasping a hand or a shoulder is a nonverbal way of communicating support.

- Keep in mind that it's okay to just sit with the patient. You don't necessarily have to have a conversation, and you certainly don't have to have "all the answers." Sometimes, just simply having someone nearby is comforting enough.

Organ Donation

Before a patient dies, he may express his wish to donate his body or body parts for medical research. Or he may wish that certain organs be surgically transplanted into other people, to help them continue their lives. Family members can also give this permission if the patient is unable to and has not made his intentions known in an advance directive.

Organ donation is another area that can involve serious emotional and ethical issues.

- The wishes of a potential donor's family may conflict with the needs of a transplant patient.
- Even if an organ is not desperately needed, controversy can arise over when to declare an organ donor legally dead.
- Since the number of organs is limited, difficult choices may have to be made about which patients should get them.

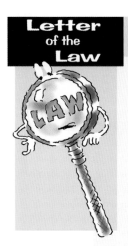

Letter of the Law

THE UNIFORM ANATOMICAL GIFT ACT

The Uniform Anatomical Gift Act of 1968 allows a person to give all or part of his body for organ transplantation or medical research. Here are the law's main provisions:

- The donor must be at least 18 years old and of sound mind.
- The body parts the donor wants to give are listed on a donor card that must be signed by two witnesses. (In many states this information can also appear on a person's driver's license.)
- A donor may revoke his consent to donation at any time.
- If a potential donor's wishes are not known, his family has the authority to donate his body or any of his body parts.
- In general, organs can be donated only to medical providers (for example, hospitals or tissue banks) or institutions (such as universities or medical schools). A donor also may name a specific person to receive a specific organ or organs.
- The recipient of a donation has the right to reject the gift.
- A donor can't be declared dead by any physician who will be involved in transplanting his organs.
- No payment of any kind may be made for an organ donation.

ORGAN HARVESTING

Harvesting organs from a deceased donor raises a difficult set of ethical issues. Some tissues and organs—such as bone, skin, corneas, and kidneys—can be taken after the patient's heart stops beating. But other organs—such as the heart, lungs, and liver—must come from a body with a "beating heart."

This raises questions about the ethics of maintaining a patient who is brain dead on life support while permission is obtained and arrangements are made to transplant his organs. If doing this is ethically acceptable, then for how long should a body be kept this way? A day? A week? Until specific organs are needed by others?

Some people are critical of organ harvesting. They believe that when a patient is brain dead, life support should stop and the patient should be allowed to die. Others believe that the benefit harvested organs can provide for those in need makes organ harvesting the right thing to do.

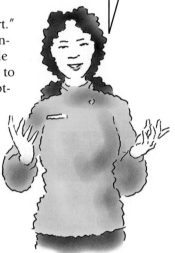

Even if a deceased patient has authorized organ donation, most physicians won't do it if the patient's family objects.

RATIONING

The number of people who need organ transplants is far greater than the number of organs available. This can raise ethical issues and controversies over who should get the organs that are available.

Medical and physical factors rule out some matches of donor and recipient.

- The donor and recipient must have compatible blood and tissue types or the recipient's body will reject the donated organ.

- The donor and recipient must be close in size and age. For example, an adult heart would not fit into the chest cavity of an infant patient.

But beyond such limitations, deciding who gets available organs can be a judgment call. This leads to some serious ethical questions about who should receive donated organs.

THIRD WORLD ORGANS

The shortage of available organs has created a thriving trade in organs from the world's poorer countries. People in these nations sell their organs or tissues for money that they desperately need to feed their families. For example, a person has two kidneys but needs only one to live. Criminals bribe hospital workers to illegally remove tissues and organs from people who have recently died.

"Organ brokers" then supply these items to waiting recipients from the world's wealthier nations. Sometimes the organ is shipped to the patient's physician for transplantation. In other cases the patient comes to the organ, or both travel to a third country for the surgery.

The buying and selling of organs is illegal in the United States, whether they come from within or outside of the U.S. In addition, every professional medical organization considers transplanting a purchased organ an unethical practice.

Cost Issues

Organ transplants are very expensive. This raises the following ethical dilemmas.

- Should only people who have insurance or are wealthy receive transplants?
- What about poor people and those without insurance? Should they get transplants, too? If so, who should pay the costs, both of the transplant procedure itself and the lifetime of anti-rejection drugs the patient must be on?

Lifestyle Issues

In 1995, a legendary baseball player who had damaged his liver through years of heavy drinking and drug abuse needed a new liver. He was also a heavy smoker and died of lung cancer soon after the transplant. Like most organs, livers are in short supply, so great controversy resulted. Serious issues of ethics arose.

- Should someone whose bad behavior destroys his own organ receive a new one when there are other people who need it, too?
- Should any patient who is dying from another disease receive a transplanted organ?

In other words, should a person's lifestyle be a factor in whether she gets an organ transplant? For example, should a heavy smoker who refuses to quit smoking receive a lung transplant, or should she be left to die from worsening lung disease? From an ethics standpoint, such questions have no easy answers.

Need Issues

The 1995 incident also raised questions about how to rank patients who are waiting for an organ to become available for transplant.

- Should the transplant list be first come, first served, or should the severity of the patient's condition determine who gets the first available organ? Should organs be awarded by lottery, in which each person has an equal chance?

- Should the recipient's age be a factor? Should younger people have priority over older people because older people will get fewer years of use from the organ?

- Should a person be moved higher on the list because she is famous, wealthy, or more "valuable" to society?

For example, should the President of the United States be moved ahead of a retired senior citizen on the transplant list if the senior citizen was registered for a transplant first? What if the senior citizen is likely to die if he doesn't receive a transplant soon?

THE ORGAN PROCUREMENT AND TRANSPLANTATION NETWORK

To manage organ donations in a fair and ethical manner, Congress created the Organ Procurement and Transplantation Network (OPTN) in 1984. A private organization, the United Network for Organ Sharing (UNOS), manages the OPTN. More than 250 hospitals across the nation are members of the UNOS. It uses the following process to match donated organs to recipients:

1. Which patients in the transplant pool have the most urgent medical need for the organ?

2. Of the patients in step 1, which have the best chance for survival after receiving the organ?

3. Of the patients from step 2, which are available immediately for surgery, both in terms of their health and their schedule?

4. Of these patients, who's been on the waiting list the longest?

The organ and patient are rushed to the nearest member hospital and the transplant surgery takes place.

WHEN THE PATIENT IS A MINOR

An extra set of problems exists when an organ donor is a child. That's because in most cases a child can't legally consent to donating one of her organs. Instead, the parents must give the consent. This raises possible ethical dilemmas for both the physician and the parents.

If the child is old enough to understand what's involved in donating a kidney to her brother, for example, she probably can give informed consent. But what if she doesn't want to do it, despite her parents' insistence on saving her brother's life? Or suppose she's too young to understand? Can the parents ethically "volunteer" this child to donate a kidney?

Choosing Between Children

Parents have a moral and legal obligation to protect the life and health of all their children. But what's more important—protecting the child who needs a kidney or protecting the health of the donor child? No transplant surgery is without risk to the donor. Plus, while the child can survive with her one remaining kidney, what if that kidney should develop problems later in her life?

Conceiving an Organ Donor

A related issue is conceiving a child in order to save an existing child. This actually happened in the 1990s. A child developed leukemia and needed a bone marrow transplant to save her life. Neither of her parents were a close-enough match for a successful transplant, and no other donors could be found. The parents decided to have a second child who could donate bone marrow to the first one.

Is having a baby to serve as a source of donated organs immoral? Does it violate the ethical principle that children should be brought into the world for their own sake and for no other motive?

INFORMED CONSENT

When a living person donates an organ, a major ethical issue is informed consent. The donor must be aware of the risks involved for him, as well as the benefits to the recipient. If the recipient is a friend or family member, a potential donor can feel great pressure to agree. If feelings of guilt or emotional distress are present, the ethics concern is whether such a donor is able to give a truly informed consent.

Fertility Issues

Some people believe that life begins at the moment of conception—when a male's sperm cell fertilizes a female's egg. Others mark birth as the beginning of life. Still others claim that life begins when heart and brain function begins—or when the child is developed enough to survive on its own, whether it's actually been born yet or not.

Another controversial issue that's related to when life begins involves the question of whether a woman has the right to prevent this process or to end it at any stage before birth. Still another issue involves the reproductive rights of persons who can't have children on their own.

ARTIFICIAL CONCEPTION

Whether or not there's a right to end a pregnancy, there's clearly no legal right to *have* children. For this reason most health plans will not pay the costs involved with enabling an infertile couple to conceive. While there may be a solid legal basis for this policy, some people question the ethics of it. They argue that since the treatments for infertility can be costly, people who can't afford them are condemned to be childless. The treatments include:

- artificial insemination
- in-vitro fertilization
- surrogate pregnancy

Some people view such procedures as miracles of medical science. Others believe them to be immoral because they violate the natural process of **procreation,** or sexual reproduction. Many religions teach that procreation is a holy event. Some religious people claim that artificial conception lessens the spiritual value of family.

Artificial Insemination

Artificial insemination is the injection of a male's sperm into a female's vagina by means other than intercourse. **AIH** (artificial insemination husband) occurs when the source of the sperm is the husband. If donor sperm is used, the procedure is known as **AID** (artificial insemination donor).

Both AIH and AID are now common practices. But legal issues can arise from each.

- What are the inheritance rights of a child conceived from a husband's frozen sperm and born years after the husband has died?
- If there's a divorce and the woman gets pregnant using her ex-husband's sperm, is he legally responsible for the child's financial support?

- What if the child of an AID wants to know the identity of her biological father? If he died a rich man, can she sue for a share of his estate?

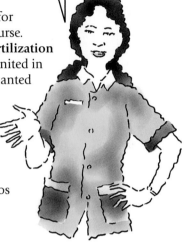

Most donor semen is tested for diseases and genetic abnormalities before it's used to impregnate patients.

In-Vitro Fertilization

Some couples have healthy sperm and eggs, but for some reason they can't conceive through intercourse. When this happens, they may turn to **in-vitro fertilization (IVF).** In this procedure, the sperm and egg are united in a test tube or Petri dish. The embryo is then implanted in the woman's uterus or frozen for later use. (**Embryo** is the medical term for a human baby in its early stages of development. From the ninth week after conception until birth, the medical term for the baby is **fetus.**)

This procedure has also produced legal and ethical controversies. For example, frozen embryos have become the subject of custody battles when couples divorce. Right-to-life issues arise when unused embryos are destroyed.

Surrogacy

If a woman can't carry a child, a surrogate can be used. A **surrogate** is a woman who agrees to carry and bear a child for a couple, usually in return for a fee. There are two types of surrogacy.

- If the surrogate contributes the egg, or is related to either the husband or the wife, it's called **traditional surrogacy.**
- If the surrogate is not related to the baby she's carrying, it's called **gestational surrogacy.**

In either case, this type of artificial conception has also raised issues. Surrogate mothers have changed their mind and have wanted to keep the baby. A surrogate mother who has contributed the egg can have a strong case for custody. Sometimes the couple has changed their minds and refused to take the baby after it is born. This often happens if the baby is born with a health problem or birth defect.

OTHER REPRODUCTIVE ISSUES

Other ethical controversies related to reproductive rights involve what some people view as the right to *not* have children. These issues center around three reproductive topics:

- **contraception**—preventing the union of the sperm and egg

THE BABY M CASE

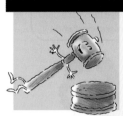

A woman signed a contract to be a traditional surrogate for a couple who could not have children. She was artificially inseminated with the husband's sperm. When she gave birth, she refused to give up the child, who became known as Baby M. Baby M's biological father and his wife sued Baby M's mother for breaking the contract. They demanded custody of Baby M.

The Verdict: The court awarded custody of Baby M to her father and his wife. But it also granted parental rights to the surrogate, because she was Baby M's biological mother. These included the right to spend time with Baby M.

- **sterilization**—surgically altering a man's or woman's reproductive organs to end the person's ability to produce children
- **abortion**—deliberately ending a pregnancy before birth

For many people, these topics involve serious moral issues. Even some people who don't oppose them on moral grounds question whether contraception, sterilization, and abortion treat children as property. If so, they ask, how ethical is that?

Legal Brief

CONSCIENTIOUS OBJECTION

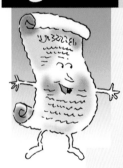

If giving or assisting in a treatment violates your religious beliefs or personal values, your employer can't make you take part in the treatment. Refusing on these grounds is called **conscientious objection.** Courts have ruled that firing an employee for conscientious objection is wrongful discharge. On the other hand, courts have supported an employer's right to transfer the employee to a different job. In either case, the responsible thing to do if you find yourself in the position of a conscientious objector is to voice your concerns before it becomes an issue. It's better to discuss your concerns openly with your employer ahead of time, rather than to walk out on a procedure in which you have been scheduled to assist.

Contraception

Contraception is more commonly known as birth control. It includes any action that a male or female takes to prevent pregnancy from occurring. These actions include:

- physical barriers, such as male condoms and female diaphragms, that block the sperm from uniting with the egg
- chemical measures, such as birth control drugs and interuterine devices (IUDs), used by the female to prevent conception
- abstinence, or avoiding intercourse either totally or around the time of ovulation (also called the "rhythm method")

Contraception has long been opposed by some religions because it prevents human life. Some people also object to contraception because they believe it encourages sexual activity among teenagers. They oppose making contraceptives such as condoms or birth control pills available to minors. Several states have laws that make the sale of contraceptives to minors illegal. However, many people today don't view contraception as a moral or ethical issue as long as adults are involved.

Sterilization

The most common forms of sterilization are vasectomies for males and tubal ligations for females. A vasectomy involves cutting the tubes that carry sperm from the testes, and a tubal ligation involves cutting the tubes that carry the egg from the ovary. Neither procedure requires hospitalization. Vasectomies can even be done in the physician's office, while tubal ligations are often done at outpatient surgical centers.

Many of the ethical issues involved with contraception also apply to sterilization. Some hospitals operated by religious organizations refuse to perform tubal ligations. This can raise questions about the ethics of such a policy if the hospital is the only one in an area.

Other ethical issues surround sterilizations that aren't elective surgeries.

- Is it ethical to require people who are mentally incompetent, or who have some hereditary disease, to be sterilized?
- Is it ethical to require women to be sterilized who are on welfare and who continue to have children?

Abortion

Abortion may be the single most controversial health care issue in the United States today. The main controversy involves human rights.

- People who support abortion argue that the privacy and ownership of one's body is a basic human right. They claim that this right gives a woman total control in deciding how to handle her pregnancy.

- People who oppose abortion argue that the right to life is also a basic human right. They claim that all abortions violate this right by ending a human life and that abortion is the same as killing a child.

A large number of issues exist somewhere between these two positions. They all involve questions of what is ethical.

- What if the woman is pregnant as a result of rape or incest? Is abortion an acceptable choice under those circumstances?

- Is it acceptable for a woman to have an abortion if tests reveal that the fetus has serious physical or mental defects? What if the defects are so severe that the child won't be able to live after it is born?

- Should a woman be able to have an abortion if continuing the pregnancy endangers her own life?

- Should a woman be able to have an abortion if the father of the fetus opposes the procedure?

- At what point in a pregnancy should a woman no longer have a right to choose abortion? Should she be able to choose abortion if the fetus is developed to the point that it could survive outside the uterus?

GENETIC TESTING

Genetics is the study of heredity—how characteristics or traits are passed from parents to offspring. The nucleus of each body cell in the human body contains 46 chromosomes. At conception, the male's sperm provides 23 of these chromosomes and the other 23 are in an egg produced by the female's ovary. The sperm and egg combine to create a cell with 46 chromosomes. This cell divides and multiplies over the next nine months to become a new person.

Each chromosome we inherit from our father and mother contains material called genes. Genes are responsible for characteristics such as eye color, hair color, and body type. Some genes are responsible for diseases that can be serious and sometimes fatal.

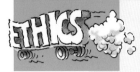

Ethics in Action | POST-PROCEDURE CARE

Every health care professional is ethically required to provide the best possible care. This means that if you oppose abortion, for example, you must set aside your feelings when caring for a patient who has had one. You can refuse to take part in procedures you find morally wrong. But you don't have a right to refuse to care for patients who've had such procedures.

Sometimes a patient will express regret after having a procedure. It's not ethical for you to force your values on her by validating her guilt. A proper response in such a situation would be, "You made the decision that you thought was right."

Medical science allows people to be tested for the presence of genes that control specific diseases. For example, such tests can tell if someone is likely to develop breast or colon cancer at some point in her life. They also can reveal that a person is carrying a gene for a fatal disease that he could pass on if he fathers any children.

Testing for the presence of such genes is also controversial. Some incurable, progressive, and fatal diseases that run in families do not develop until a person reaches middle age.

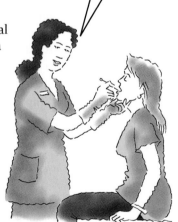

Collecting samples for genetic tests is easy. Blood, saliva, and tissue cells all provide good materials for testing.

- Some people with a family history of a disease want to be tested to see if they have the gene. They want to know their prospects for the future, so that they may plan their lives.

- Other people whose relatives have died from an incurable hereditary disease may choose to not be tested. Since the disease is incurable, they'd rather live their lives assuming they are not affected than know for sure if they're going to get it.

Prenatal Testing

Some parents choose to genetically test their unborn children during pregnancy. The most common test is **amniocentesis.** The physician uses a needle to withdraw a small amount of the

Legal Brief   GENETIC DISCRIMINATION

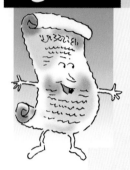

Since genetic testing has become more accurate and wide-spread, so has **genetic discrimination.** This is unequal treatment of people based on their genetic makeup. Some health and life insurance companies, adoption agencies, and others have discriminated against people who are at risk for certain hereditary diseases.

- Nearly all states now have laws that prevent health plans from discriminating based on the results of genetic tests.
- Most states now have laws barring genetic discrimination in employment.
- The federal Health Insurance Portability and Accountability Act (HIPAA) prohibits health insurers from denying coverage based on a person's genetic information.
- The federal Americans with Disabilities Act prohibits employers from discriminating against an employee with a genetic disease.

fluid that surrounds the child in the mother's uterus. The fluid is then tested for the presence of genetic defects such as Down syndrome, a condition that causes retardation.

Prenatal genetic testing has become quite common. But it raises a number of difficult ethical issues.

- If a woman is carrying a child who will be severely impaired, is abortion an acceptable option? On the other hand, do children whose disabilities will make their lives difficult and painful have a right to be born?
- Should a fetus be tested for genetic disorders that may show up only later in life? Would a positive test for such a disease justify an abortion? What if the test is not 100 percent accurate?
- If prenatal testing reveals a disease the parents are not aware they are carrying, and that may strike one or both of them in later life, should they be told?
- Should a woman have the right to abort a healthy child only because it doesn't have the genetic traits (for example, gender or eye color) the parents desire?

Legal Brief BABY DOE LAWS

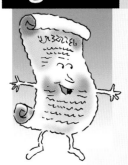

In the past, legal and ethical controversies have arisen when parents chose to withhold life-saving treatment from premature babies born with severe disabilities. As a result, many states passed what are called Baby Doe laws. These laws require treatment in such cases. They also allow providers to be prosecuted for withholding it.

People who support Baby Doe laws view the controversy as a right-to-life issue. Opponents believe that such laws ignore quality-of-life issues. They also claim that Baby Doe laws are an example of a mistaken belief that laws should take the place of ethical decision making.

Testing Newborns

As many as five percent of children are born with a **congenital disorder.** This is an illness or other condition that is present before birth. For this reason, it's common practice in many hospitals to do genetic tests on all newborns.

Also nearly all states have laws that require newborns to be tested for phenylketonuria (PKU), so that treatment can begin at once if the test is positive. Left untreated, PKU can cause severe mental retardation and even death.

These genetic tests may also reveal if the man listed on the birth certificate as the baby's father is actually not related to the child at all. Data suggest that this may be the case in as many as ten percent of births. The ethical dilemma: should one or both parents be told?

Biomedical Research

Many of the medical advances you've read about in this chapter have resulted from years of research. This research often has included experimentation on human subjects to perfect new drugs or treatment techniques. Other research has focused on altering human genes to accomplish certain goals:

- to cure medical conditions
- to keep hereditary diseases from being passed on
- to ensure that desirable traits will appear

CLINICAL TRIALS

Many physicians take part in **clinical trials,** or medical research involving human subjects. Drug companies often sponsor and pay for these trials when they are testing the safety or effectiveness of a new drug.

A clinical trial can take place at many sites, involving scores of physicians and hundreds of subjects. Sometimes, some or all of a physician's subjects may come from among the patients of her medical practice.

Informed Consent

A patient's participation in a clinical trial must always be voluntary. It's also important that patients who choose to take part do so with informed consent. This requires that the following information be provided to the patient.

- What's being studied and why? For example, if the study involves a new drug, what's the drug supposed to do? Is it being tested to find out if it works, to determine the dose that's effective, to see if it's safe, or to discover the side effects it may cause?

- What are the risks involved in taking part? How likely is each risk to occur, or is that even known at this point in the research?

- What benefits might be expected? Not all medical research directly benefits the subjects being studied.

- How is the study designed? For example, is there a control group who will not receive the drug or treatment, but a harmless pill or procedure instead? Are subjects assigned to the treatment group or the control group at random, or can the physician choose which patients go in which group?

- Is the study "blind?" In other words, will the patient know whether he's in the treatment group or the control group? Will the physician know?

The physician must explain all this information, even if it means the patient may decide not to participate in the study. Patients should be encouraged to weigh the answers to all these questions before agreeing to take part.

The Ethics of Clinical Trials

Some people question the ethics of using a control group when conducting medical research. These subjects will not benefit from the study. Patients with the condition being studied who are in the control group will therefore get no treatment for their

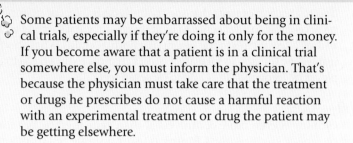

MEDICAL ASSISTANTS AND CLINICAL TRIALS

Some patients may be embarrassed about being in clinical trials, especially if they're doing it only for the money. If you become aware that a patient is in a clinical trial somewhere else, you must inform the physician. That's because the physician must take care that the treatment or drugs he prescribes do not cause a harmful reaction with an experimental treatment or drug the patient may be getting elsewhere.

condition. Even those in the treatment group may suffer if the treatment proves not to be effective.

Blind studies raise special concerns because even the physician may not be aware whether a patient who needs treatment is actually getting it. In any case, a physician has an ethical responsibility to advise a patient whose condition worsens to withdraw from the study and return to proven treatment. If the condition is life threatening, the physician has a responsibility to advise the patient to remove herself from the study. The only exception is if the study is the only hope the patient has for a cure.

GENETIC ENGINEERING

Genetic engineering involves altering people's genes to cure or eliminate genetic diseases or to change genetic traits. It's been done with plants and animals for many years to produce better quality livestock and disease-resistant crops. Crops have also been genetically engineered to increase their food value or to enable them to grow in harsher climates.

Genetic engineering in humans is still in its early stages. However it holds great hope for the future. At the same time, it offers the possibility of creating a "super race," a possibility that many people find ethically troubling.

Gene Therapy

Gene therapy is treatment that occurs from altering or eliminating a harmful gene. It's becoming an effective method for preventing, correcting, or treating certain diseases. For example, a person's genes could be altered to deal with a hormone deficiency or to allow the body to better absorb certain therapeutic treatments. Normal copies of genes could be inserted into people's cells to replace genes that cause certain diseases or disorders.

Gene therapy raises many ethical questions and issues. Some people worry that its use could go beyond correction and prevention to creation of traits that society finds desirable. For example, if it's acceptable to alter genes to fight dwarfism, what's wrong with adding a few inches to the height of a normal child? What about using gene therapy to increase a child's chances to be a basketball player by "growing" the child to be seven feet tall?

Cloning

Cloning is even more controversial than gene therapy as a form of genetic engineering. **Cloning** is using a single cell from an organism to grow an exact copy of that organism.

Science is continuing to perfect the techniques of cloning. As research continues, more complex organisms are being cloned. Animals that have been successfully cloned include mice, cats, monkeys, and farm animals such as sheep, goats, pigs, and cattle. The meat of cloned farm animals can now be purchased in grocery stores. So can the milk from cloned cows.

Besides providing a steady source of high-quality meat, cloning can encourage production of animal organs and tissues for medical use. For example, valves from a pig's heart can be transplanted to replace damaged or diseased valves in a human heart.

Supporters claim that providing these benefits makes cloning ethically acceptable. Some opponents object to the ethics of using animals in this way, while others fear the long-term effects of cloning on the human race.

The United States banned the cloning of human beings in 2000. But other countries continue to allow the cloning of human embryos for research purposes. Supporters of this research claim that infertile couples could someday have children that were genetically related to them. Furthermore, they see cloning as a source of "spare parts" for existing humans. Opponents of cloning find such ideas ethically troubling.

Most days I'm so busy that I wish I had a clone!

Stem Cell Research

Stem cell research is another hugely controversial area of genetic engineering. **Stem cells** are the "master cells" from which the body generates specialized cells. They are the building blocks that scientists think could be used to create new organs and tissues that would allow the body to heal itself.

The controversy over stem cell research is less about this prospect, however, than it is about the research itself. That's because most stem cells used in the research come from human embryos, though some types of stem cells do come from cells of adults. Opponents of embryonic stem cell research object to what they view as the destruction of human life for scientific research.

Supporters of stem cell research argue that the embryos used to get stem cells would be discarded anyway, even if they were not used for research. Opponents do not find this argument convincing, however. Recent advances have allowed stem cells to be harvested from umbilical cords of new babies and even from adults. Researchers hope that these new techniques will make their work less controversial.

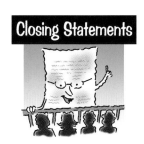

Closing Statements

- Bioethics deals with what's "right" in issues of life and death. Some of the bioethical issues involved in the practice of medicine include when life begins and ends, organ donation, reproductive rights, medical research, and genetic engineering.

- Patients have a right to die. That right includes the right to refuse treatment. If the patient is not able to make that decision, then the physician, in consultation with the patient's family, must decide what's best for the patient. Some patients write advance directives that indicate their wishes and instructions for care in case they're ever in a situation in which they can't speak for themselves.

- Many people choose to donate organs at their death, or even while they're still alive. Organ donation raises ethical issues and questions about when organs should be taken and who should receive them. Special concerns apply when the organ donor is a minor. The shortage of available organs makes these ethical issues all the more important and controversial.

- Reproductive rights are especially controversial. Artificial conception includes artificial insemination, in-vitro fertilization, and surrogacy. For some people, these means of having children raise issues of morality and violation of natural procreation processes. The prevention of procreation through contraception, sterilization, and abortion involve right-to-life and right-to-privacy issues that are also highly controversial.

- Genetic testing and genetic engineering can identify and correct a variety of conditions, sometimes even before a person is born. Despite the good that some people feel comes from such advances, other people view them as unnatural and immoral. Still others raise concerns about their possible misuse, especially when gene therapy or cloning is involved. Stem cell research is among the most controversial genetic engineering topics. Like many of the others, it raises right-to-life issues for some people.

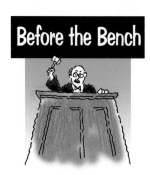

Before the Bench

Answer the following multiple choice questions.

1. An advance directive is a written statement of a patient's
   a. level of care that allows the patient to be comfortable.
   b. list of organs to be donated after his death.
   c. desired time and date to end his own life.
   d. treatment wishes if the patient is not able to state his wishes at the time

2. Which document provides the most freedom of choice in dealing with a patient's end-of-life issues while the patient is still able to make decisions for herself?
   a. a living will
   b. a health care proxy
   c. an informed consent
   d. a durable power of attorney

3. What is the *first* stage of the grieving process?
   a. anger
   b. denial
   c. sadness
   d. none of the above

4. What is the *final* stage of the grieving process?
   a. sadness
   b. bargaining
   c. acceptance
   d. none of the above

5. Which is *not* true of organ donations made through the Uniform Anatomical Gift Act?
   a. If a donor's wishes are unknown, his organs can't be donated.
   b. A donor may donate organs to a medical provider or name a specific person to receive an organ.

c. A donor can't receive payment for donating an organ.

d. A donor can revoke his consent to donate at any time.

6. Which of the following is used to prevent pregnancy?
   a. artificial insemination
   b. contraception
   c. in-vitro fertilization
   d. surrogacy

7. Amniocentesis can be unethical if it's used to screen for
   a. Down syndrome.
   b. eye color.
   c. Huntington's chorea.
   d. hemophilia.

8. Which of the following is part of the debate over the morality, ethics, and legality of abortion?
   a. the right to privacy
   b. the right to life
   c. basic human rights
   d. all of the above

9. What's the *most important* factor in conducting an ethical clinical trial?
   a. There should be some value or benefit to each person who takes part in the study.
   b. The clinical trial should be a blind study.
   c. All who take part give a fully informed consent.
   d. Participants should be assigned to the treatment group or to the control group randomly.

10. The area of genetic engineering that *currently* offers the *most* benefit to human health is
    a. gene therapy.
    b. cloning.
    c. stem cell research.
    d. surrogacy.

GLOSSARY

abandonment   the situation in which a physician withdraws from a contractual relationship with a patient without proper notification while the patient still needs treatment [Chapter 2]

abortion   expulsion of the product of conception before the fetus can be viable and live outside the uterus [Chapter 10]

abuse   in medical billing, billing for services that were provided but were unnecessary; contrast with *fraud* [Chapter 5]

accessory   a person who does not actually commit a crime, but contributes to the commission of a felony (called *an accessory before the fact*); a person who knows that a felony has been committed and aids or conceals the offender (called *an accessory after the fact*) [Chapter 2]

accommodation   the process of adapting or adjusting, especially by a compromise or convenient arrangement, with another party in a dispute [Chapter 9]

accreditation   official authorization or approval that a person or institution meets the standards needed to conduct certain tasks [Chapter 5]

administrative law   the branch of law that involves government agencies and the rules they create [Chapter 2]

administrative rules   regulations created by government agencies that watch over certain practices or professions; violation of regulations can bring disciplinary penalties or even prosecution under criminal law [Chapter 2]

advance directive   a document such as a living will or durable power of attorney in which a patient expresses his or her wishes regarding health care prior to a critical medical event [Chapter 10]

affirmative action   measures designed to favor people who are at a disadvantage because of their race, gender, or some other factor, particularly by improving their employment or educational opportunities [Chapter 8]

affirmative defense   a denial of guilt or wrongdoing based on new evidence rather than simple denial of a charge [Chapter 4]

AID (artificial insemination donor)   an artificial insemination procedure in which a donor's sperm is used; also see *artificial insemination;* contrast with *AIH (artificial insemination husband)* [Chapter 10]

AIH (artificial insemination husband) an artificial insemination procedure in which the sperm of the woman's husband or partner is used; also see *artificial insemination;* contrast with *AID (artificial insemination donor)* [Chapter 10]

amniocentesis the insertion of a needle through the abdominal wall and into the uterus of a pregnant female to obtain amniotic fluid in order to examine the fetal chromosomes for abnormalities and to determine the sex of the fetus [Chapter 10]

anesthetic a drug that temporarily blocks transmission of nerve conduction to produce a loss of sensation and sometimes loss of consciousness [Chapter 3]

arteries vessels that carry blood from the heart to tissues throughout the body; contrast with *veins* [Chapter 3]

artificial insemination the introduction of sperm into the female reproductive tract by other than by natural means; also see *AID, AIH,* and *in-vitro fertilization (IVF)* [Chapter 10]

assumption of risk a doctrine that a person may in advance accept the chance of being injured and relieve another person of the requirement to act with due care; an affirmative defense that the plaintiff cannot receive compensation for injuries from the defendant because the plaintiff knowingly assumed the risk of injury [Chapter 4]

autopsy an examination of a dead body, usually with dissection and examination of vital organs, to determine the cause of death [Chapter 6]

avoidance the act of deliberately avoiding the occurrence of something, such as an action or a dispute; preventing something from happening [Chapter 9]

beneficence the state or quality of doing good, especially performing acts of kindness and charity [Chapter 1]

best interest standard an ethical principal to guide physicians in making treatment decisions for incompetent patients that involves determining what action would be in patient's best interests in a particular situation [Chapter 10]

bioethics a field of study that deals with the moral implications of biological research and applications, especially in medicine [Chapter 1]

borrowed servant doctrine an exception to the doctrine of *respondeat superior;* borrowed servant doctrine releases an employer from liability for an employee's actions if the employee is working for someone else; contrast with *respondeat superior* [Chapter 4]

brain death   the lack of any activity in the central nervous system as indicated by a flat electroencephalogram (EEG) [Chapter 10]

breach   the failure to perform a duty that is required by law or by an agreement [Chapter 3]

breach of contract   the failure, without good reason, to fulfill one's duties or obligations under a contract [Chapter 2]

capitation payment   a predetermined, per-person payment made to a physician by a managed care group, such as an HMO, in return for medical care provided to enrolled individuals; also see *health maintenance organization (HMO)* and *managed care* [Chapter 6]

case law   a body of law that has been established by judicial decisions in court case—as distinguished from law created by legislation or by administrative rule [Chapter 2]

cause   a reason or justification for an action, such as terminating an employee [Chapter 8]

cause of action   the grounds (legal reasons or basis) that entitle a plaintiff to bring a lawsuit [Chapter 8]

catheter   a tube that is inserted into canals, vessels, passageways, or body cavities for diagnostic or treatment purposes, to allow injection or withdrawal of fluids, or to keep a passage open [Chapter 3]

certification   a voluntary process, usually involving testing, establishing that a person meets a certain standard of competency in a particular professional area; contrast with *license* and *registration* [Chapter 5]

charting   documenting or recording information in a patient's chart, or medical record; also see *documentation* [Chapter 7]

civil law   branch of law that applies to private rights and disputes between persons; contrast with *criminal law* [Chapter 2]

clinical trial   a scientifically controlled study of the safety and effectiveness of a treatment, such as a drug or vaccine, by using consenting human subjects [Chapter 10]

cloning   a process by which an organism is created without procreation, usually from a single cell of the parent organism, to create an identical copy of the parent organism; contrast with *procreation* [Chapter 10]

collaboration   the act of working together with someone to produce or accomplish something [Chapter 9]

common law   the body of law that is based on customs and general principles, including case law, that is applied in situations that are not covered by statute law [Chapter 2]

communicable disease   a disease that can be transmitted by contact with an affected individual or the individual's discharges, or indirectly by another agent (such as an insect) that carries the disease from one organism to another [Chapter 6]

comparative negligence   determination of liability in which damages may be divided among multiple comparative defendants; negligence is measured according to the degree of its contribution to the injury (often in percentages); also see *negligence* and *contributory negligence* [Chapter 4]

compassion   pity for the sufferings of others that makes one want to help them; also see *empathy* and *sympathy* [Chapter 4]

compensation   something, usually an amount of money, that is given to make up for a loss; also see *compensatory damages* [Chapter 3]

compensatory damages   money awarded to a defendant to compensate him or her for losses suffered as a direct result of the injury suffered; contrast with *punitive damages* [Chapter 2]

competition   striving for a goal in rivalry with another [Chapter 9]

complaint   the initial action that starts a lawsuit and that the plaintiff's allegations against the defendant and sets forth the plaintiff's demand for remedy [Chapter 2]

compromise   a settlement of a dispute in which each party gives up some demands so that an agreement can be reached that satisfies all sides to some extent [Chapter 9]

conflict   a serious disagreement that arises from differing, competing, or opposing persons, interests, or ideas [Chapter 9]

congenital disorder   a condition that exists at or dates from birth and that was acquired during development in the uterus and not through heredity [Chapter 10]

conscientious objection   a person's refusal to do something because he thinks it is morally wrong [Chapter 10]

conspiracy   an agreement between two or more people to commit an illegal act [Chapter 5]

contingency   a fee for a lawyer's services that is paid only on the successful completion of the services and that is usually calculated as a percentage of the gain obtained for the client [Chapter 4]

continuing education   an instructional program that brings participants up to date in a particular area of knowledge or skills [Chapter 5]

contraception   the practice of or methods used to prevent pregnancy as a result of sexual intercourse [Chapter 10]

contract   an agreement between two or more parties in which each party agrees to do something; also see *expressed contract* and *implied contract* [Chapter 2]

controlled substance   any substance that is strictly regulated or outlawed because of its potential for addiction or abuse [Chapter 5]

contributory negligence   negligence by the plaintiff that contributed to the injury at issue, but was not the sole cause of the injury; also see *negligence* and *comparative negligence* [Chapter 4]

copayment   a fixed fee that some health insurers require a patient to pay at the time a medical service is provided or when filling a prescription [Chapter 5]

creed   a set of beliefs or opinions, especially religious beliefs [Chapter 9]

criminal law   public law that deals with crimes and their prosecution; contrast with *civil law* [Chapter 2]

culture   the beliefs, social institutions, customs, and arts shared by a people in a place or time [Chapter 1]

custodian   an individual entrusted with guarding and keeping the property of or having custody of another person [Chapter 7]

damages   the amount of money a court orders a defendant to pay the plaintiff when the case is decided in favor of the plaintiff; also see *plaintiff, defendant, liable, compensatory damages,* and *punitive damages* [Chapter 2]

data bank   a large storage of information held in a computer [Chapter 5]

defendant   the party against whom a criminal or civil legal action is brought [Chapter 2]

deposition   a pretrial statement made under oath by a party or witness in a legal action in response to oral or written questions and cross-examination [Chapter 2]

dilemma   a situation requiring a choice between two or more unpleasant or undesirable alternatives [Chapter 1]

discipline   training that corrects behavior and enforces control, obedience, and order [Chapter 8]

disclose   to reveal or expose to view [Chapter 7]

discovery   the required disclosure of facts or documents relevant to a civil of criminal action; the process by which a party to the action obtains information held by the other party [Chapter 2]

discrimination   unequal treatment when there is no reasonable distinction between those treated favorably and those treated unfavorably, especially if the treatment is based on race, religion, gender, disability, or some basis other than individual merit [Chapter 8]

dismissed   a judge's decision to reject court consideration of a complaint; also removed from a position or fired [Chapter 2]

docket number   the number assigned to identify a case on a list of legal actions to be heard by a court [Chapter 7]

doctrine   a principle or position in a branch of knowledge or system of belief, especially a principle of law established by previous court decisions; also see *precedent* [Chapter 3]

doctrine of professional discretion   a legal principle that allows a physician not to allow a patient to view his medical record if the physician believes that something in the record might cause the patient harm if he sees it [Chapter 7]

documentation   the preparation or assembly of written records; also, the act of recording an event in a document, as in a patient's medical record, in order to have a record of the event; also see *charting* [Chapter 7]

Drug Enforcement Administration (DEA)   an agency of the federal government that is empowered to enforce laws and regulations regarding the purchase, administration, and use of controlled substances; also see *controlled substance* [Chapter 5]

due care   the care that an ordinarily, reasonable, and prudent person would use under the same or similar circumstances [Chapter 5]

durable power of attorney   a legal document that gives a person the authority to make medical decisions for a patient if the patient is not in a condition to make those decisions himself; also see *health care proxy* and *living will* [Chapter 10]

duty of care   a legal responsibility to use due care toward others in order to protect them from unnecessary risk of harm; also see *due care* [Chapter 3]

elective procedure   a treatment that is beneficial but not essential for a patient's survival [Chapter 6]

electronic medical records   information about patients that is recorded and stored on a computer [Chapter 7]

emancipated minor   a person under the age of majority who's is legally considered free from the custody, care, and control of his or her parents; also see *minor*; contrast with *mature minor* [Chapter 6]

embryo   a developing organism from fertilization to the end of the eighth week; contrast with *fetus* [Chapter 10]

emergency   a sudden, serious situation that requires immediate action [Chapter 4]

empathy   the ability to imagine, share, understand, and be sensitive to the feelings and problems of another person; also see *sympathy* and *compassion* [Chapter 1]

employment-at-will   a legal doctrine under which an employer or an employee can end employment at any time and for any reason that is not contrary to law [Chapter 8]

endorsement   the process by which a state automatically licenses a professional from another state whose credentials meet its own licensing requirements; contrast with *reciprocity* [Chapter 5]

ethics   guidelines for moral behavior that are set by religious beliefs, professions and other groups in society, and by individuals themselves; compare to *medical ethics* and *professional ethics* [Chapter 1]

etiquette   the rules and standards for correct and polite behavior in society or among members of a profession [Chapter 1]

euthanasia   deliberately bringing about the death of a person who's suffering from an incurable disease or condition, either actively (by administering a lethal drug) or passively (by withholding treatment); also known as mercy killing [Chapter 10]

expert witness   a person whose knowledge, skill, training, or experience qualifies him or her to provide testimony to aid a jury or judge in matters that exceed the knowledge of the average person [Chapter 2]

expressed consent   a statement of approval from the patient for the physician to perform a given procedure after the patient has been educated about the risks and benefits of the particular procedure; also see *informed consent*; contrast with *implied consent* [Chapter 6]

expressed contract   a formal agreement, stated orally or in writing, between two or more parties; also see *contract*; contrast with *implied contract* [Chapter 2]

federal laws   statutes or administrative rules passed by Congress or created by a regulatory agency of the executive branch of the national government [Chapter 2]

fee-for-service   the traditional practice of billing a patient or the patient's health insurance plan for treatment and other services that were provided [Chapter 6]

fee splitting   an unethical and sometimes illegal practice that involves the sharing of fees between physicians for patient referrals [Chapter 5]

felony   a grave crime for which the punishment may be imprisonment for more than a year [Chapter 2]

fetus   a developing organism from ninth week after fertilization to birth; contrast with *embryo* [Chapter 10]

fidelity   faithfulness and loyalty to someone or something [Chapter 1]

fraud   any act, expression, omission, or concealment that is designed to deceive another to her disadvantage; in medical billing, fraud is billing for services that were not provided; contrast with *abuse* [Chapter 5]

gatekeeper   a health-care professional (usually a patient's primary care physician) who regulates the patient's access to hospitals and specialists in order to manage the care and control the costs of treating the patient; also see *primary care physician* [Chapter 6]

gene therapy   the insertion of purposely altered genes into cells to replace defective genes in the treatment of genetic disorders, or for a disease-fighting function such as the destruction of tumor cells [Chapter 10]

genetics   a branch of biology that deals with the heredity and variation of organisms [Chapter 10]

genetic discrimination   the different treatment of individuals because of their actual or presumed genetic differences; also see *discrimination* [Chapter 10]

genetic engineering   techniques used to separate and rejoin genetic material (especially DNA) and to introduce the result into an organism in order to change the organism's characteristics [Chapter 10]

gestational surrogacy   a form of surrogacy in which the surrogate is not genetically related to the fetus; contrast with *traditional surrogacy* [Chapter 10]

good faith   honesty, fairness, and lawfulness of purpose, with no intent to defraud, act maliciously, or take unfair advantage [Chapter 5]

Good Samaritan law   a state law that protects off-duty physicians and sometimes other health care practitioners from liability when offering care in emergency situations [Chapter 5]

gross   flagrant or extreme, especially in offensiveness [Chapter 8]

health care proxy   a person authorized to make health care decisions for another; a document that gives a person such authorization; also see *durable power of attorney* and *living will* [Chapter 10]

health maintenance organization (HMO)   a type of insurance that provides comprehensive health care to members through contracted physicians, with limited referral to outside specialists and paid for by fixed payments determined in advance; contrast with *preferred provider organization (PPO)* [Chapter 6]

honesty   the quality of being truthful, sincere, and direct; also see *integrity* [Chapter 1]

hostile workplace   a form of sexual harassment that interferes with the victim's work performance or creates an offensive working environment that affects the victim's psychological well-being; also see *sexual harassment;* contrast with *quid pro quo* [Chapter 8]

humility   the quality of being humble, or having a modest opinion of oneself and one's own importance [Chapter 1]

implied consent   informal approval from the patient to medical treatment that is not directly stated but instead indicated by signals, inaction, or silence; contrast with *expressed consent* and *informed consent* [Chapter 6]

implied contract   an agreement between parties, such as a patient and a physician, that is not stated but is assumed from the actions of the parties; contrast with *expressed contract*; see also *contract* [Chapter 2]

incapacity a lack of ability to do something [Chapter 5]

incident report a formal document that provides a detailed account of events about an accident, treatment mistake, or other unusual event; serves as a factual statement of the event in case of a lawsuit [Chapter 4]

informed consent a statement of approval from a patient, often given in writing, to perform a given procedure after the patient has been educated about its benefits and risks; also see *expressed consent*; contrast with *implied consent* [Chapter 4]

integrity the quality of being honest and having strong moral principles; also see *morals* and *honesty* [Chapter 1]

internship a period of practical hands-on training; in the medical profession, a physician's first year of training after graduating from medical school and before she has passed the examination required to obtain a license to practice medicine; contrast with *residency* [Chapter 5]

intentional torts deliberate wrongful acts that cause injury or harm to another; also see *tort*; contrast with *unintentional torts* [Chapter 3]

interrogatories written questions, required by law to be answered, that one party in a lawsuit directs to the other party to obtain information as part of the discovery process; also see *discovery* [Chapter 2]

in-vitro fertilization (IVF) the mixing in a laboratory dish of sperm with eggs that have been surgically removed from an ovary, followed by the implanting of one or more of the now-fertilized eggs into a female's uterus [Chapter 10]

just cause behavior that provides grounds to terminate an employee; a behavior that provides the basis for a legal action [Chapter 8]

justice the quality of being reasonable and fair; right and fair behavior [Chapter 1]

kickback the money that is paid to someone who has helped another to make a profit, often illegally [Chapter 5]

law of agency a doctrine holding that when one party acts on behalf of and under the control of a second party, the second party is liable for the actions of the first party as long as the first party's actions are within the scope of their relationship; also see *respondeat superior* [Chapter 4]

laws formal rules to guide conduct or actions that must be followed and that are enforced by a government authority; also see *administrative law, case law, civil law, common law, federal law, public law,* and *private law* [Chapter 1]

liable   obligated to, bound to, or answerable for something under the law [Chapter 4]

libel   a false and malicious written statement aiming to damage a person's reputation or character; contrast with *slander* [Chapter 2]

license   permission granted by a government to engage in some occupation or action that is unlawful without such permission; contrast with *certification* and *registration* [Chapter 5]

life support   the treatment and equipment needed to keep a seriously ill or injured patient alive without which the patient would not survive [Chapter 10]

living will   a document in which the signer indicates preferences or directions for the administration, withdrawal, or withholding of life-sustaining medical treatment in the event of terminal illness or permanent unconsciousness; contrast with *durable power of attorney* and *health care proxy* [Chapter 10]

malfeasance   the commission of a wrongful or unlawful act that involves or affects the performance of one's duties [Chapter 3]

malpractice   negligence, misconduct, lack of ordinary skill, or a breach of duty in performing a professional service and that results in injury or loss [Chapter 3]

managed care   a system that is designed to control the costs of health care through managed programs in which the physician accepts limits on the amount charged, and sometimes on the services performed, and the patient is limited in the choice of physician; also see *health maintenance organization (HMO)* and *preferred provider organization (PPO)* [Chapter 6]

Material Safety Data Sheet (MSDS)   a federal government-required document that provides information on the risks, safe handling, storage, and treatment for exposure to each hazardous chemical or other hazardous material present in a workplace [Chapter 8]

mature minor   an unemancipated minor who under state law can make his or her own medical decisions in certain circumstances, usually involving requests for birth control or psychological evaluation or treatment for pregnancy, drug or alcohol abuse, or sexually transmitted diseases; also see *minor* and *emancipated minor* [Chapter 6]

Medicaid   a program of medical care designed for those unable to afford regular medical service and financed jointly by the state and federal governments [Chapter 5]

medical ethics   the moral principles and standards of conduct that govern or influence the practice of medicine; also see *ethics* and *professional ethics* [Chapter 1]

medical record the record of a patient's medical information, such as medical history, care or treatments received, test results, diagnoses, and medications taken [Chapter 7]

Medicare a government program of medical care that provides and partially pays for medical care for persons age 65 and over and certain people with disabilities [Chapter 5]

misconduct unacceptable behavior, especially by a professional person [Chapter 8]

minor a person who has not reached the age of majority—the age at which a person is granted by law the rights and legal responsibilities (such as the ability to sue or to be bound by the terms of a contract) of an adult; in most states the age of majority is age 18; also see *emancipated minor* and *mature minor* [Chapter 6]

misdemeanor a crime that is punishable by a fine and a term of imprisonment of less than one year, and that is not served in a penitentiary [Chapter 2]

misfeasance the performance of a lawful action or an official duty in an improper or unlawful manner [Chapter 3]

morals principles of right and wrong that form a person's standards for behavior [Chapter 1]

motion an application made to a court or judge to obtain an instruction, an order, or a ruling [Chapter 2]

negligence the failure to exercise the care that would be expected from a person of ordinary caution in a similar situation in protecting someone else from a foreseeable and unreasonable risk of harm [Chapter 3]

nonfeasance the failure to do something that should be done, especially something that a person has a duty or obligation to do [Chapter 3]

oncologist a physician who specializes in the treatment of tumors, especially cancerous tumors [Chapter 3]

overwriting an electronic process that wipes a computer's hard drive clean and prevents recovery of previously deleted files [Chapter 7]

palliative care care that eases pain and other discomfort without curing the underlying disease or condition [Chapter 10]

paraprofessionals trained aides who assist a medical professional [Chapter 5]

participating providers the physicians, hospitals, and other health care providers who are part of a preferred provider organization (PPO); also see *preferred provider organization (PPO)* [Chapter 6]

peer review a process by which a professional's colleagues review and judge his actions [Chapter 5]

perseverance continued, steady effort, especially to achieve an objective or goal [Chapter 1]

personal ethics a person's guidelines for acceptable behavior that result from his or her own individual morals and values [Chapter 1]

phantom billing in medical billing, billing for services that were never performed [Chapter 5]

plaintiff the party who institutes a legal action or claim [Chapter 2]

policy manual a collection of written statements that explain a business's practices, standards, and goals in basic areas of operation; in a medical office, these areas would include policies related to patient privacy, clinical treatment, patient communications, and documentation; contrast with *procedures manual* [Chapter 4]

precedents earlier judicial decisions that ordinarily must be followed by a judge when deciding a similar case; also see *doctrine* [Chapter 2]

preferred provider organization (PPO) a type of health insurance that provides health care to members by giving them economic incentives to use certain contracted physicians, laboratories, and hospitals that have agreed to supervision and reduced fees; contrast with *health maintenance organization (HMO)* [Chapter 6]

premises a building or part of a building, usually with its surroundings [Chapter 4]

primary care physician (PCP) the physician who is responsible for directing all of a patient's medical care and deciding whether that patient should be referred to a specialist; also see *gatekeeper* [Chapter 6]

private law a branch of law concerned with private persons, property, and relationships; contrast with *public law* [Chapter 2]

privileged communication a statement made by one person to another who is in a confidential relationship with that person (such as a doctor-patient or attorney-client relationship); privileged communication generally cannot be required by law to be revealed to a third party [Chapter 6]

procedures manual a collection of written, step-by-step instructions for every task performed in an institution; in a medical office, a procedures manual should contain a separate written procedure for each clinical and administrative task; contrast with *policy manual* [Chapter 4]

procreation reproduction; the bringing forth of offspring, usually by means of sexual intercourse; contrast with *cloning* [Chapter 10]

professional courtesy   the practice of treating other physicians and their families, or other health care professionals, for a reduced fee or free of charge [Chapter 6]

professional ethics   the moral principles and standards of conduct that govern or influence the practice of a profession and the behavior of persons who work in that profession; also see *ethics* and *medical ethics* [Chapter 1]

progressive discipline   a system of increasingly severe penalties and other steps designed to correct an employee's negative behavior rather than terminating the employee [Chapter 8]

property right   a claim of ownership [Chapter 7]

prosecution   in a criminal action, the process of seeking formal charges against a party and pursuing those charges to judgment in a court of law; the party who brings a criminal action against another party; also see *prosecutor* [Chapter 2]

prosecutor   a government attorney who presents the state's case against the defendant in a criminal trial [Chapter 2]

public law   the area of law that deals with the relations of individuals with the government and regulates the organization and conduct of society and government; a law passed by a legislature that affects the general population of a territory; contrast with *private law* [Chapter 2]

punitive damages   money awarded to the plaintiff in cases of serious or malicious wrongdoing, to punish the defendant and discourage others from behaving in the same way; contrast with *compensatory damages* [Chapter 2]

quality improvement (QI)   a program undertaken by a health care organization to achieve or maintain certain specified standards in the delivery of patient care [Chapter 4]

qui tam   a legal action brought by a person (the *whistleblower*) on behalf of a government against someone alleged to have violated a statute, especially one against defrauding the government through false claims; also see *whistleblower* [Chapter 5]

quid pro quo   a form of sexual harassment in which the satisfaction of sexual demands is made on the condition of job benefits or continued employment, or is used as the basis for employment decisions about the individual; also see *sexual harassment*; contrast with *hostile workplace* [Chapter 8]

reasonable person standard   a legal doctrine that judges a person's actions in a situation according to what a rational person would have done in the same situation [Chapter 3]

reciprocity   the process by which a license granted by one state may be accepted in other states by prior arrangement between those states; contrast with *endorsement* [Chapter 5]

registration   a credentialing process that indicates that a person has met certain professional standards of an occupation; contrast with *certification* and *license* [Chapter 5]

regulations   rules and restrictions that are intended to control something [Chapter 2]

residency   a period of hands-on training in primary care or a medical specialty that a physician undertakes after graduating from medical school and passing the licensing examination; contrast with *internship* [Chapter 5]

res ipsa loquitur   a legal doctrine stating that things do not have to be explained beyond the obvious facts and that a person is presumed to be negligent if she had control over what caused an injury, even if there is no specific evidence of an act of negligence [Chapter 3]

res judicata   a legal doctrine stating that a matter settled in court cannot be raised again; it exists to protect parties in a case that has already been decided [Chapter 4]

respondeat superior   a legal doctrine that makes an employer liable for the wrongdoing of an employee if it was committed within the employee's scope of employment; also see *law of agency* [Chapter 2]

responsibility   the quality of being able to be relied on to carry out important duties [Chapter 1]

revoke   to take back a grant of permission, such as a license, especially because of misconduct; contrast with *suspend* [Chapter 5]

scope of practice   the range of activities as defined by state law that a health care professional is certified or licensed to perform [Chapter 3]

seminar   a meeting of a relatively small group of people to discuss or study a topic under the guidance of an instructor; also see *workshop* [Chapter 5]

settle   to conclude a lawsuit by an agreement negotiated between the parties, usually out of court [Chapter 7]

sexual assault   sexual contact with a person without his or her consent, or that is inflicted on a person who is incapable of giving consent (because of age or physical or mental incapacity) or who places the assailant (such as a physician) in a position of trust [Chapter 8]

sexual battery   intentional and offensive physical sexual contact with a person who has not given or is incapable of giving consent [Chapter 8]

sexual harassment   unwelcome verbal or physical sexual conduct directed at another person, especially an employee or coworker, because of gender or sexual orientation [Chapter 8]

slander   false oral statements that damage a person's reputation or character; contrast with *libel* [Chapter 2]

standard of care   how most other health care providers with similar training would handle a patient's care under similar circumstances [Chapter 3]

stare decisis   the doctrine under which courts follow precedent (prior court decisions) on questions of law in order to insure consistency and stability in the administration of justice; the doctrine holds that departure from precedent is permitted only for compelling reasons, such as to prevent the creation of injustice [Chapter 2]

statute of limitations   a time limit for a certain legal action to be taken; for example, the maximum length of time in which a patient may file a lawsuit [Chapter 2]

statutes   laws enacted by the legislative branch of a government [Chapter 2]

statutory law   the body of law that consists of laws enacted by a legislature [Chapter 2]

stem cells   unspecialized cells (generally embryonic cells) that have the potential to become any type of body cell [Chapter 10]

sterilization   a procedure that deprives an organism of the power to reproduce; also, a process that kills microorganisms by the use of physical or chemical agents [Chapter 10]

subpoena   a written order requiring the person upon whom it is served to appear in court or face a penalty for failure to comply [Chapter 2]

subpoena duces tecum   a subpoena that commands someone to produce specified evidence that is in his possession [Chapter 7]

substituted judgment test   an ethical principal that guides physicians in making treatment decisions for incompetent patients by asking what decision the patient would make if she were able [Chapter 10]

summary dismissal   a judge's dismissal of a court action, such as a lawsuit, without the usual full legal procedures [Chapter 8]

surrogate   someone or something that serves as a substitute for another; in medicine, a woman who agrees to carry and bear a child for a couple, usually in return for a fee; also see *gestational surrogacy* and *traditional surrogacy* [Chapter 10]

suspend   to take away temporarily a permission or privilege, such as a license; contrast with *revoke* [Chapter 5]

sympathy   a feeling of sorrow or pity for someone that results from sensitivity to their problems or situation; also see *empathy* and *compassion* [Chapter 1]

technical defenses   defenses in a lawsuit that are based on principles of law rather than on the actions of the defendant [Chapter 4]

telemedicine   the practice of medicine in which the doctor and patient are separated and that involves the use of two-way voice and visual communication, such as by satellite, computer, or closed-circuit television [Chapter 6]

terminal disease   a disease or illness that leads to death, especially a slow death, and that cannot be cured [Chapter 10]

terminally ill   having a disease or illness that leads to death [Chapter 10]

tolerance   the practice of recognizing and respecting the beliefs or practices of others; the ability and willingness to endure someone or something without complaining [Chapter 1]

tort   a wrongful act (other than a breach of contract) that injures another and for which the law imposes civil liability; a violation of a duty that is required by law, rather than by contract, and for which damages or other relief may be obtained [Chapter 2]

tortfeasor   a person who commits a tort, or a wrongful act [Chapter 3]

traditional surrogacy   a form of surrogacy in which the surrogate contributes the egg or is genetically related to one parent of the fetus she is carrying; contrast with *gestational surrogacy* [Chapter 10]

Tri-Care   a government program that provides health care to members and retirees of the U.S. military and their families [Chapter 5]

unbundling   the practice of submitting an insurance claim with several separate CPT procedure codes rather than a single code that covers all those services; sometimes done deliberately (and illegally) in order to obtain a larger payment [Chapter 5]

unintentional torts   accidental actions that cause harm to a person or property; also see *tort*; contrast with *intentional tort* [Chapter 3]

upcoding   an illegal billing practice that includes billing for services more complex than those that were actually performed, billing for brand-name drugs when generic drugs were administered, or listing treatment for a more complicated diagnosis than the patient presented with [Chapter 5]

unemployment compensation   payments of money made to unemployed workers, chiefly by state governments, to help pay expenses until they find another job [Chapter 8]

values professional or personal moral standards and principles of behavior; compare to *morals* [Chapter 1]

veins the tubular branching vessels that carry blood from the body's tissues toward the heart; contrast with *arteries* [Chapter 3]

vendor a person or company who sells something [Chapter 9]

verdict the decision of a jury on one or more matters submitted to it in a trial; in civil actions the verdict is a finding for the plaintiff or for the defendant, and in criminal actions is the verdict can be guilty or not guilty [Chapter 2]

vital statistics statistical data that relate to births, deaths, marriages, public health, and disease [Chapter 6]

waive to voluntarily give up a right, claim, or privilege under law; to refrain from enforcing or requiring something [Chapter 6]

warrant a court-issued document that gives someone legal authority to do something, such as a search warrant or an arrest warrant [Chapter 7]

whistleblower an employee who brings wrongdoing by an employer or other employees to the attention of a government or law enforcement agency and who is usually protected by law with rights and remedies in the event of retaliation; also see *qui tam* [Chapter 5]

workshop a brief and intensive educational program for a small group of people that focuses especially on techniques and skills in a particular field; also see *seminar* [Chapter 5]

wrongful discharge the termination of an employee for illegal reasons or for reasons that are contrary to public policy—for example, for refusing to take part in an unlawful activity [Chapter 8]

INDEX